DISEASES OF THE LIVER.

THE

Diseases of the Liver:

JAUNDICE, GALL-STONES, ENLARGEMENTS, TUMOURS, AND CANCER:

AND THEIR TREATMENT.

BY

J. COMPTON BURNETT, M. D.

———

Second, Revised and Enlarged Edition.

———

"Das ist eben das wahre Geheimniss, das
Allen vor Augen
Liegt, euch ewig umgibt, aber
von Keinem gesehen."

Schiller.

B. JAIN PUBLISHERS (P) LTD.
NEW DELHI-110055

Printed in India

Price: Rs. 40.00

Reprint Edition **2003**

© Copy right with Publishers

Published by:
B. Jain Publishers (P) Ltd.
1921, Gali No. 10, Chuna Mandi,
Paharganj, New Delhi-110055 INDIA

Printed in India by :
J.J. Offset Printers

ISBN 81-7021-367-3
BOOK CODE B-2113

PREFACE TO FIRST EDITION.

———

TO those accustomed to treat diseases
of the liver with remedies having an
elective affinity for the organ itself, the
contents of this volume must appear more
or less self-evident. I refer more particularly to the practitioners of scientific
therapeutics usually called homœopaths.
But the practitioners of traditional medicine will find in my pages a great deal to
interest them, and not a little that is new;
new at least to them.

Those of my readers who have a
taste for the more strictly doctrinal part
of my subject, I would refer to my small
work entitled "Diseases of the Spleen and
their Remedies Clinically Illustrated," to
which this is intended to be a companion
volume.

The prevailing ignorance of good organ-remedies is lamentable. Not long since a lady came to me for a chronic liver affection of nine years' standing, and, though her physician is a man of high standing in the profession, and a doctor of medicine of the University of London, his sole treatment had consisted in giving the accursed morphia to lull the pains. He had never even tried one single good organ-remedy, and this notwithstanding the fact that patient has long been profoundly jaundiced. And this, too, is I fear, a fair sample of the everyday work of the men of light and leading in the profession.

The pain being the outcome of the disease, the treatment should have been directed to the causal complaint, and not to the effect—the pain. Had this been done, the lady would, in all probability, have been cured of the fundamental disease; as it is, her disease has become formidable, and probably incurable, and she herself is a hopeless, helpless, will-less morphia eater.

It is in the hope of throwing a little light into this dismal darkness that these pages are sent to the Press.

October 2, 1890.

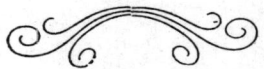

PREFACE TO SECOND EDITION.

THE first edition of this work being exhausted, this second edition gives me an opportunity of saying by way of one word, that my little treatise "Diseases of the Spleen" contains much that, in justice to my subject, ought to have appeared in "Diseases of the Liver," I refer more particularly to the theoretical considerations on the place of organopathy in the homœopathic edifice. Attention was called to this, but most of my reviewers have clearly overlooked the point and hence it has come to pass that I feel that my dear little bantling has not had quite fair play. It has, so to speak, been dotting about the world on one leg much to my parental concern.

My stand-point in *Diseases of the Liver* is a scientific and doctrinal one and one moreover of great practical importance and my little book is not merely an *omnium gatherum* of **hepatic** odds and ends. For my justification I now add *Part I,* which ought **to have** appeared in the first edition.

J. COMPTON BURNETT, M.D.

86 Wimpole Street,

London, W.

Midsummer, 1895.

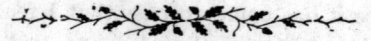

To the Memory

.OF

Rademacher

THE RESUSCITATOR OF
PARACELSIC ORGANOPATHY

THESE PAGES ARE GRATEFULLY DEDICATED

BY

The Author.

PART I.

The Autonomy and Hegemony of the Organ in the Organism : Being Remarks Introductory to the Cure of Organ Diseases by Organ Remedies in Reference to Diseases of the Liver.

The Diseases of the Liver:

The Automomy and Hegemony of the Organ in the Organism.

THE interaction of the human organism with its environment has generally been recognized in every age according to the views current at the time, the relations of the microcosm to the macrocosm used to be a big chapter in medical doctrine.

That man acts upon his environment has been well demonstrated by the changes that have been wrought in physical nature in the United States, Canada and Australia since they have become inhabited. The differences in the American, Canadian, and Australian shew clearly that nature reacts back on man who is moulded and formed by his climate. I am personally acquainted with a gentleman, now resident in London, who at twenty years of age left England for Eastern Europe, and there remained till he was thirty years of age when he returned to this country. When he went he had an abundance of light curly hair. On his return his hair was abundant and curly but nearly *black*, so that his own mother did not know him and his own brother who went on board the steamer by which this gentlemen returned and hunted for him amongst the passengers entirely failed to recognize him though he stood close by him for some time, he was looking for a light-haired man. After ten years further residence in England his hair had almost returned to its original light color.

When the spermatozoön and the ovule meet and marry their inter-action comes to a complete organic union resulting in a new organism, thus of dual origin, and finding a suitable habitat in the womb sets up a connection with the mother. Here the maternal organism and the fœtus interact with one another: the influence of the fœtal organism upon the mother's organism is very curious: her breasts grow, her back widens, her shoulders broaden, her gait alters. Yet not-

2

withstanding the dependence of the fœtus upon the mother and the maternal changes upon the fœtus the two lead independent lives and may even have certain diseases independently of one another.

In this way we come up to what we may conceive to be the nature of the physiological position of the various organs of the body to the organism itself; what the macrocosm is to the microcosm that the microcosm is to the separate organs.

Although the crasis of all the fluids of the body and the stroma of all its organs and parts must in the main be about the same, both physiologically and pathologically, still there is a certain individual life and equality being inherent in each organ and part and I surmise that there are many *kinds* of blood corpuscles.

For the present, confining ourselves to the organs only, we wish to enquire somewhat into the question of how and how far a given organ is to be considered therapeutically apart from the organism of which it forms a part and without which it has no existence.

This idea has swam more or less before my mind for many years, and I have given expression to it in several of my writings, particularly in my "Diseases of the Spleen" and in the second part of this work, and its importance in my daily clinical work increases with time.

The question of the independent
existence of the organ, or rather of
the existence of *a something in each
organ* (and I believe in each region
and part) deserves the most careful study and consideration because
of its bearing upon treatment, and
upon the question of the dose, viz:
whether to use high, low or me-
dium dilutions, and this quite apart
from organotherapy.

On this peculiar something in
each organ the Rademacherian
practice of medicine is largely based
but nothwithstanding its practical
utility it has thus far not been
scientifically elucidated so little indeed that but few regard it as of
any particular importance; in fact,
we may say that it has barely any

recognized existence at all. And yet there it is, and for a number of years has been of so much help to me in my clinical work that I feel impelled to dwell upon the subject here a little more at large. Brown-Séquard's work in the later years of his life has physiologically taught us that there is in the very deed a real "self" in each organ and that such organ has a functional importance for its organism to whose entirety it belongs. The effects of spaying and castrating are well known and really prove the point so far as ovaries and testicles are concerned—this has been recognized all along. The old doctrine of signatures is laughed at by almost all physicians, inclusive of the homœopaths,

and yet it is not without considerable foundation in fact; and, indeed, facts in great numbers may
be drawn from homœopathic liter-
ature in support of its real practical
value. It has often helped me and
I have long since ceased to ridicule
it. Of course, it can easily be
turned upside down and made to
look silly, but still there it is and
in the long run will most certainly
be justified by science. I am very
certain Hahnemann believed in it
for it is manifest that he drew very
numerous indications from it for
his remedies. That Constantine
Hering also believed in it seems
pretty certain, and Hering knew
his Hohenheim, of whose works he
made a splendid collection. Von
Grauvogl, too, shows that he was

not uninfluenced by it. Rademacher ever made merry over it, and yet many of his remedies came into use through it, *Chelidonium* to wit. Von Grauvogl years ago recommended *Pulmones vulpecularum* in asthma and I have followed his recommendation with advantage, he was laughed at a good deal at the time, but now science comes along and puts a stop to the ridicule so long cast upon Paracelsic organ feeding.

There is a peculiar disease consisting in an enlargement of the hands and feet, face, head an extremities, called Marie's Disease, or Acromegaly, with which and enlargement of the pituitary gland— is commonly associated—here it would appear that the nutrition of the extremities is directly influenced by the pituitary gland. The enlargement of the pituitary gland is said to be a true hypertrophy of its substance and not a neoplastic process.

That the influence of the pituitary gland affects development and nutrition is also shewn by the other overgrowth and undergrowth tendencies connected with pituitary disease.

The autonomy and hegemony of the individual organ is even more clearly demonstrated by modern research in regard to the thyroid gland.

As is well known Goitre, or Derbyshire neck, is exceedingly

common in Switzerland. Some dozen years ago Dr. Kocher, of Berne, communicated to the German Surgical Congress the results of a hundred extirpations of Goitre and shewed that there arose in some of his observations an affection consecutive to the total ablation of the thyroid gland which he described as *cachexia strumipriva.* In English medical language struma is synonymous with scrofula while botanists understand by struma the swelling or protuberance of any organ. In Central Europe struma is used as a synonym of Derbyshire neck and of other not necessarily strumous swellings.

The next step was the recogni-

tion of the similarity of the artifact cachexia strumipriva with the
idiopathic malady known as myxœdema and reasoning that inasmuch as as the artifact disease
arose in consequence of the total
ablation of the thyroid it might be
that myxœdema was likewise due
to a lack of the thyroid organ-
influence on the organism. Feeding the myxœdematous with ani-
mal thyroids soon shewed that the
reasoning was sound, and this
nutritional therapeutics is now the
recognized treatment of myxœdema
due to simple thyroid atrophy.
And very pretty it all is.

Kocher finding that the total
ablation of the thyroid led to myxœdema afterwards modified his

mode of operating and adopted the
plan of leaving a portion of the
gland capable of functional activity
instead of totally ablating it. And
he tells us that he has since operated on 900 cases of Goitre in this
manner and in no case has any
cachexia strumipriva supervened.
Furthermore, Kocher has hunted
up a number of his old cases of
total ablation in whom the cachexia
had appeared and fed them with
thyroids with the most satisfactory
results.

It has been found that overfeed-
ing with thyroids acts poisonously
upon the organism generally and
specifically, and this will no doubt
be called thyroidism, if it has not
already received that name.

Lanz and Trachewski have made experiments with thyroid feeding under the immediate supervision of Kocher himself and produced in dogs *"tous les symptomes de la maladie de Basedow,"* and what is positively startling *"ce mode de traitement peut* amener à la longue une *atrophie complète des parties saines de la glande thyroide" ! !*

Now, the fates are distinctly unkind to our allopathic friends who had begun to score one by their cure of myxœdema with thyroid glands added to the food of the sufferers: the place of the atrophied thyroid being supplied by the thyroid food, and here comes experimental science and shews that the thyroid feeding in the long run contingently produces atrophy and not only atrophy, but *complete* atrophy of the healthy parts of the thyroid gland. So that in future the dose of the thyroid extract must be lessened because this new therapeutic acquisition of allopathy over which we homœopaths had certainly become not a little jealous, is after all not only pure homœopathy but its symptomatic and pathologic homœopathicity is demonstrated all ready for us in their own laboratories. Now our allopathic friends must do as they did in regard to tuberculinum, viz: admit the efficacy of small doses and with it the truth of the homœopathic law, or officially drop the thyroid business, as they did with tuberculinum. They will go out of the thyroid business in time confused by their own work, because without the light of the homœopathic law it must end in confusion. So after all Paracelsus was right in recommending his lung-to-lung and kidney-to-kidney homœopathy, and the dignity of the organ has risen to university rank and fellowship.

What I in this volume am really concerned with is the importance of the organ, its complete autonomy and hegemony, as bearing on the diseases of the liver.

The functions of the liver are too large a chapter for me now to touch upon, but the newest data of science in regard to goitre and thyroid feeding bring out into a clear light these points:—

1. That the organ in the organism does indeed possess not only autonomy but hegemony, *i. e.* the organ is an independent state in itself and in and on the organism exercises an important influence.

2. That both a plus and a minus of a given organ results in disease of the organism.

3. That the organ-to-organ homœopathy of Paracelsus is a scientific fact.

And we thus see that organ-remedies by restoring the disturbed organ to health cures the organism itself.

I have for years fought for the

recognition of the organ in the organism from the clinical side and maintained that organopathy lies at the very root of homœopathy in its simplest and most elementary form, and now that orthodoxy is officially proclaiming "organo-theraphy" (Paracelsic organ-to-organ homœopathy) and now that physiologists firmly and faithfully believe that all the glands have a creative, formative, directing, controlling, nutritive, antitoximal internal secretion, surely I need fight no longer the cause of the organ in the organism.

By the way, it seems to me that Hale's *Law of Dose* is amply confirmed by the clinical results of organotherapy, the law may not be of universal application but it and it only, explains many of the phenomena of homœopathic cures. Iron produces plethora and anæmia and who amongst us can deny the splendid cures of anæmia by iron in full dose? We all see them daily. And who would for a moment think of using full doses of iron in plethora? and certainly we use with much advantage infinitesimal doses of iron for many symptoms of plethora.

We may say that the full doses are nutritional only, but it seems to me that that is not all. The newer facts of organotherapy, presently to come may, perhaps, clear the matter up.

PART II.

The Diseases of the Liver:

Jaundice, Gall-stones,

Enlargements, Tumours, and Cancer,

and their Treatment.

JAUNDICE.

IF anyone shall maintain that Jaundice is not a *greater* disease of the liver, but a minor one, I shall reply, Then such a one has never had the curious complaint. Jaundice was the indirect efforts at independent thought in medicine; it was in this wise:—A student was working with Professor H——-

with the microscope while he had a bad cold in his head—in the hot trickling dewdrop stage—and finding that microscopizing under the circumstances was not an easy matter, he said to his professorial friend, "What's good for a cold in the head?"

"Oh," said he, "sniff up cold water into your nostrils—that'll cure it quickly."

Studiosus set his microscope aside; went home. Once there, forthwith sniffed cold water most diligently into his nostrils, and *cured* the said coryza there and then. A sweet cure! as the sequel shewed.

The next day he had the beginning symptoms of catarrhal jaundice, and in two days the affection
was well-established.

Professor H. was again consulted, and said he must give up
hospital work at once, and take a
holiday in the hills.

Being conversant with all the
facts of the case, it occurred to me
that as catarrhal jaundice was due
to a catarrh of the gall-ducts, just
as the coryza was a catarrh of the
nose, so if we could only get at the
gall-ducts as readily as at the
nostrils, we might wash them out
also, and thus *cure* the jaundice, as
the coryza had been cured.

I have had a certain number of colds in the head to treat during the years that have since elapsed, but I have never recommended Professor H.'s plan of sniffing cold water into the nostrils, believing a catarrh of the nose to be less bad than a corresponding state of the gall-ducts. This simple narration really touches at the very foundations of *all* curing: The young man was not well; nature sought to rid his organism of something harmful to his organismic self; she set up a watery discharge from a small portion of the mucous lining of the body, near the surface and not otherwise too much functionally occupied. This hot

running from the nose was really
a curative expression of the organism. (The young man had been
long living and working in the
most foul atmosphere of dissecting
rooms and hospital wards.) The
cold water *stopped* it (the flux, not
the disease,) and then nature fell
back upon the liver, as she so often
does.

*Centrifugal fluxes and discharges
should not be lightly stopped.*

Why **the** flux? *Whence* the discharge? Let the questions of the
why? and whence? be answered as
we go along. Here I merely insist
upon the elementary truth that a
morbid process having a, perhaps,
time-honored name, may be never-

theless no disease at all, but merely a means of cure set up by nature herself, and that there are diseases which it is disadvantageous or dangerous to cure, that is to cure in the sense in which the verb to cure is commonly used in English by the thoughtless. Of course to effect a *really* radical cure of any *primary* disease can never be other than a gain to the individual.

CASE OF CATARRHAL JAUNDICE CURED BY *Chelidonium majus.*

A good many years since I was summoned to see a country gentleman for sudden indisposition. It was a rather tedious railway journey, and a humble friend of the family, anxious to enlighten me, told me that the squire had the " *Yeller Janders.*" Yellow the patient was, indeed, and the colour was from jaundice ! There were the usual symptoms—constipation, scanty urine of a dark yellow browny colour, and debility with depression of spirits. *Chelidonium majus* in small material doses, put matters right in a few days, leaving the patient, however, weak.

" What medicine have you been giving my husband ?"

" A new remedy."

" What's it's name."

" *Chelidonium majus.*"

" What's the English of that ?"

" The greater Celandine."

" Then it is not by any means a *new* remedy, for it is in my old Herbal, in which it is recommended for jaundice."

And so it was: the use of the greater Celandine in jaundice has trickled down to us through the ages from the primary source of the doctrine of signatures.

Of *Chelidonium majus*, I would say that it is in this country the greatest liver medicine we have aud there is, in all conscience, no lack of hepatics. Some of my early success in practice was due to my use of *Chelidonium.*

It came about thus: I went to see an important lady for a well-known physician in the north, he being too busy to attend, but said lady strongly objected to new doctors. She took a look at me— as I subsequently learned—from a position where she herself was invisible to me, and did not like the look of me. So I was sent away with many apologies from the daughter. Her hepatalgia was easier just at that moment: she would wait till her own physician would come.

A few days later the pain in her right side became unbearable, and said physician again sent me. This time I was admitted and found her in very great pain in the hepatic region: she had had it at intervals for very many years—about thirty years, if I remember rightly. The liver was very much enlarged and the pains very acute; there was no jaundice, the tongue mapped.

I mixed some *Chelidonium majus* and had it given pretty frequently: it eased the pain more promptly than ever the pain had been relieved before, and finally cured it altogether. Her whole life was changed. To make amends for having refused to see me on my first calling upon her she presented me with a piece of plate, and sent me subsequently very many of her suffering friends.

So *einflusserich* was this venerable dame that I feel her practical influence to this very day.

This cure, and its gratifying results to a struggling young doctor, fixed my attention a good deal upon *Chelidonium*, and upon liver affections, which are everywhere so common; and it has been my lot to relieve or cure a very large number of liver diseases—and from this wide experience I now write.

My first real acquaintance with *Chelidonium* was from Dr. Richard

Hughes's " Pharmacodynamics," a work to which I owe so much, and which I sincerely commend to all who wish to understand the actions of drugs.

I would not be too sure of my botanic knowledge, but I have an idea that *Chelidonium* is the only plant, indigenous to this country, which possesses a yellow juice. That the colour of this juice led to its use in liver diseases on the lines of the doctrine of Signatures the historically competent will hardly deny. That it has a specific affinity for the great gall-organ anyone may verify for himself if he will take a few drachms of the mother tincture in divided doses. It is kindly and gentle in its action, which action is fully set up with only a very minute dose, but inasmuch as my more intimate knowledge of it comes to me from the Rademacherians, I have generally used it in small material doses.

It will be interesting to give Rademacher's experience with *Chelidonium.*

He used it as an organ remedy, or in other words on the homœopathic principle in its elementary form of specificity of seat.*

---

* I have entered so fully into the question of the identity of the organopathy of the Hohenheimians and the specificity of seat of the homœopaths, in my work entitled "Diseases of the Spleen and Their Remedies Clinically Illustrated" that I may fairly refer my readers hereto in lieu of going over the same ground again here.

4

RADEMACHER'S USE OF
Chelidonium.

Rademacher, with the charming simplicity of really great knowledge, tells us in regard to *Chelidonium*, that he had long despised it is worthless, and confessedly to his shame, for he remarks that it was a celebaated hepatic remedy in olden times. (See his *Erfahrrungsheillehre*, p. 163.)

He then enters into a long dissertation upon its action and comes to the conclusion that it affects the "inner liver." He says a physician need have no great experience to know that the disease of the liver, that in its perfected form shews itself as jaundice, has endless gradations that in every-day life and in medical speech are not regarded as jaundice. Still the very slightest degree of the jaundice-affection shews itself in the urine by its pale gold colour, and in the skin, particularly in that of the face, by its more or less dirty look. And where there is but little gall in the motions and no icteric discolouration of the skin, it follows that we have in such cases to deal with not merely an obstruction to the outflow of the gall into the duodenum, but with that unknown organ by which the gall is prepared from the blood; this gall-making organ is ill so that bile is

4

not duly prepared at all, and therefore none can be either poured out or absorbed into the skin, or cast out by the urine. This is what Rademacher calls the "inner liver," not indeed as an anatomical expression, but as a figure of speech to convey to the mind a more or less accurate and concrete conception of the sphere of action of the *Chelidonium majus*.

This conception of the true sphere of action of *Chelidonium* is, I think, correct.

The cases cited by Rademacher are mostly "bilious fevers."

Where the gall ducts are alone implicated he considers *Nux vomica* the right remedy. Hence *Cheli-*

aonium would be indicated in alcholia as well as in jaundice when the affection is primary to the "inner liver."

Rademacher's favorite mode of using it is the simple juice of the plant with just as much alcohol as will clarify and preserve it. His dose was at one time one scruple of his tincture a day, but in chronic cases of liver affections he subsequently came down to two or three drops a dose, given four or five times a day. He even came down to one-drop doses diluted in half-a-cupful of water, till at last he thinks he might be accused of copying the homœopathic posology of "Mr. Hahneman!" He tells us

however, ("*Erfarhrungsheillehre*,"
p. 176), that he first appreciated
the curative value of small doses
from Helmont,* who roused in his
soul the thought that *small doses
of drugs might have great curative
effects*.

But Rademacher confesses that
he at first did not clearly perceive
the importance of the small dose
until he had got rid of his earlier
and more gross views, and came
from diligent observation to get
concise views of primary organ-
diseases as they really exist in
nature. In a foot-note (p. 176)
he protests that the small dose cannot be correctly spoken of as

---

* *Opera omnia*, p. 552, in the chapter with the
superscription *Butler*.

"homœopathic," but as being the
property of Paracelsus, and refers
to the eleventh chapter of the fifth
book of Hohenheim's "Chirurg-
ische Schriften," *De Causis et
origine luis Gallicæ*, which he recommends his readers to peruse at-
tentively, and concludes thus . . .
"wenn sie dieses gethan, werden
sie wol nicht mehr von homöopathischen Arzeneigaben sprechen,
sondern sie werden begreifen, dass
die Wahrheit—*unwäg und unmess-
bare Arzeneigaben können, wenn
das durch Krankheit veränderte
Verhältniss des Körpers zur Aus-
senwelt sich dazu eigene, wunder-
volle Heilwirkungen äussern*—mit
der sogenannten homöopathischen

Theorie gar nicht in Berührung kommt."

In other words . . . unweighable and unmeasurable doses of remedies can produce wonderfnlly curative effects when the condition of the body in regard to its environment have been altered by disease and thus rendered susceptible thereto, and thus have nothing at all to do with the so-called homœopathic theory.

But this only by the way, I am writing of the Diseases of the Liver; still it is pretty evident that Rademacher in his later days had become conscious that his own practice and teachings were

leading him, nilly-willy, homœo-
path-wards.

CASE OF ENLARGEMENT OF THE LIVER WITH JAUNDICE CURED BY *Chelidonium*.

A lady of seventy, stout, and given to very little exercise, came under my observation, and on examination I found her severe and frequent right-sided pains were due to a swelled liver, which was tender in pressure. Skin and conjunctivæ subicteric, motions containing but very little bile; urine on the contrary loaded with it. She was at the seaside and this it was, she said, that had upset her liver. Tongue coated, giddy, low-spirited, pulse intermittent, insomnia, lethargic, loss of appetite, fear of death.

Chelidonium majus in small material doses resulted in complete recovery in ten days, when she returned home with a regular pulse, clear eyes and skin, and all the functions normal, and very decidedly of opinion that life, even at seventy years of age, is not at all a bad thing.

ENLARGED LIVER AND CONGESTION OF THE RIGHT LUNG, CURED BY *Chelidonium.*

A young officer in the Army was invalided home from India for liver and lung disease and came to me.

I found his liver large and tender, the right lung engorged, his skin very muddy, bowels costive, and he was dreadfully depressed and weak. He was quite sure he was in consumption. The lung affection I regarded as consecutive to the engorgement of the liver, there being, in the words of Rademacher, a primary affection of the "inner" liver. *Chelidonium* in small material doses quite restored him to health in three weeks. In due course he returned to his regiment.

CASE OF PRONOUNCED JAUNDICE CURED BY *Chelidonium*.

A middle-aged gentleman, a merchant, returned from the East Indies with very severe jaundice, which had resulted in considerable emaciation. The voyage home and a stay of some duration in the north had not mended matters. He was very depressed in spirits, almost the colour of mahogany, and the urine was very scant and brown-yellow. His bowels very constipated.

How quickly and pleasantly he was cured, he even now never tires of telling his Manchester friends.

I might tell of a lady who had severe and long-lasting jaundice and who was speedily cured by *Chelidonium*, and of a notable number of other cases of liver affections cured by it, but it is needless. What I have already narrated will suffice.

I would, however, just dwell upon the fact that *Chelidonium* will very frequently cure engorgements of the right lung even when it is a concomitant of true phthisis, but it has no influence over the general phthisical state, other than what pertains to, and results from, the lower half of the right lung and liver. As an intercurrent remedy in the hepatic complications of phthisis it is capable of rendering important service.

Likewise as an intercurrent remedy in gall-stones it is useful, as is also *Myrica cerifera*, but both stand far behind *Hydrastes* in this affection.

My own conception of its true seat of action is that it affects the liver cells : Rademacher's "inner" liver.

There are numerous affections of the liver that *Chelidonium* will not touch curatively at all, and therefore it must not be regarded as a liver cure-all, which it is not.

For instance, it affects the left lobe of the liver much less than does *Carduus Mariæ*, to a consideration of which we will proceed after having first given a short account of Rademacher's use of a combination of *Chelidonium* and *Calcarea muriatica*.

RADEMACHER'S USE OF *Chelidonium* AND *Liq. Calcariæ muriat.*

Our author tells us he is convinced that there exists in nature a liver disease that can only be cured by a mixture of *Chelidonium* and *Liq. Calcariæ muriat.*

This is his formula:—

> ℞   Liq. Calcariæ muriat., ʒii.
>
>   Tinct. Chelidonii,   ʒi.
>
> M.

He administered fifteen drops in half-a-cupful of water five times a day. With this he cured many cases of grave fevers and hepatic affections that did not mend with either remedy by itself, but he tells us he knows of no reliable or characteristic indications for its choice.

I might add that muriatic acid once had a seemingly well-founded reputation as a liver remedy; and some still esteem it highly.

The Curative Sphere of *Carduus Mariæ* in Liver, Spleen, and Abdominal Affections.

Certain remedies have very limited special spheres of influence and our power to cure diseases is largely conditioned by our knowledge of such spheres. I am increasingly impressed with the importance of knowing *where* the remedy acts by special elective affinity. As I have dealt with spleen affections by themselves, without making any special reference to *Carduus mariæ* (the seeds are the officinal part), I will at once exemplify its action here.

ENLARGEMENT OF LIVER AND SPLEEN CURED BY
Carduus.

A young lady, of sixteen sum-
mers, was brought to me by her
mother on the seventh of Septem-
ber, 1887, for severe attacks of
vomiting that had lasted for three
months. She was often roused
rudely from her sleep in the morning with an attack of vomiting.
Her constitution had been dam-
aged by diphtheria, and eighteen
months previously she had had
varicella. I treated the case symp-
tomatically with great relief to the
vomiting, but the pains in the
5

abdomen became rather worse than better.

After I had given her my old favorite *Nat. mur.* 6 she was still further improved, but there the thing still was: I had relieved the symptoms but I had not cured the real primary seat of the same.   I then did what might with advantage have been done before the treatment was begun, viz: I made a careful physical examination of the bare epigastrium and of the two hypochondria.   With what result?   The note in my case book taken at the time will enlighten us . . . . "Liver and spleen both very much enlarged so that they seem almost to fill the abdomen."

Here I had to do with the severe
and long-lasting vomiting which
yielded partially to close symptomatic treatment but would not
get quite well . . . . (Oh, how
often are we in this unsatisfactory
state); and a physical examination
revealed the reason of my failure.
I had treated the case with remedies that were homœopathic to the
superficial symptoms, but NOT
homœopathic to the cause of those
symptoms; the degree of homœopathicity was not adequate though
it went a long way towards it.

Here I fell back upon my Rademacherian experience with *Carduus* and gave five drops of the
matrix tincture in a tablespoonful

of water, night and morning, and this cured the enlargement both of Spleen and of Liver, and as this enlargement was the cause of the pains and vomiting, of course pains and vomiting likewise disappeared.

The only further abnormality which I could discover in the young lady after taking the *Carduus mariæ* for about five weeks was an indurated condition of a few of the cervical glands of her left side: the side on which she had been vaccinated; *Thuja occidentalis* 30, in infrequent doses, cured these and patient has had no vomiting or any of its concomitants since. She continues well to date.

Although my own prescription

of *Carduus* was from pure experience, there can be hardly any doubt that an adequate proving would shew its homœopathicity to the case, inclusive of the enlargements of liver and spleen.

Riel's proving of *Carduus* shews it to produce pathogenetically: "nausea, uneasiness, pain, vomiting, with inflation of the abdomen, &c."

The generally improved appearance of the young lady after she had been a month under the *Carduus* was very striking, and repeatedly remarked upon, by friends who were not acquainted with the circumstances of her ill-health and its treatment at all.

The *kind* of liver enlargement which *Carduus* cures is in the transverse measurement.

By way of comparison I will now quite shortly exemplify the *kind* of enlargement of the liver which is cured by *Chelidonium*; it will be seen that the comparison is crude and mechanical, yet withal, I submit, not without practical value.

ENLARGEMENT OF THE LIVER IN THE PERPENDICULAR LINE CURED BY *Chelidonium.*

An independent gentlemen of thirty, usually resident in Paris, came over to London to consult me in the early part of the year 1886, and that for his liver and for dyspepsia. He had twice had jaundice in previous times. His symptoms were waterbrash, indigestion, constipation, attacks of intra-abdominal chilliness; he was very dusky, his urine had a strongly urinous smell. His liver reaches almost up to the right nipple.

An ounce of the tincture brought the liver back to the normal; the dose was five drops in water, two or three times a day, and sometimes once a day. But altogether he consumed nearly an ounce.

This is the *kind* of hepatic enlargement which *Chelidonium* rights in small material doses. But it did not restore the patient to complete health; why? For the simple reason that the increase in the perpendicular measurement of the liver was only a *part* of his complaint, the other bearings of the case being foreign to my present thesis. Suffice it to say that his liver was cured by the *Chelidonium*, and patient continues well

in these (and now in the other) respects to the present time.

It is well to realize that an organ-remedy while capable of curing an organ-disease, and all the concomitant symptoms which *arise from* the organ-disease, nevertheless can in the nature of things *not* cure the concomitant symptoms in the patient when these symptoms stand in no nexus with such organ-disease. Thus I treated a young lady for a liver disease and gave her successively *Carduus*, *Chelidonium*, *Natrum sulphuricum*, *Taraxacum*.

She had a mapped tongue and vomiting, with headaches and squinting. The liver was reduced to its right dimensions and the vomiting was cured, but the mappiness of the tongue remained, and patient did not *feel* well. But the tongue became normal after a month of *Thuja* 30 She had headaches which she herself termed bilious and the others neuralgic, and there was a third kind of headache called by another name and which seemed distinctly connected with the squinting. The bilious headaches ceased after the use of the before-mentioned hepatics; the neuralgic headaches continued till after the *Thuja*, and disappeared simultaneously with the mapped state of the tongue. The squint-headaches she still gets, and remedies like *Glonoin* and *Gelsemium* do them good

From these considerations it is manifest that there are cases that cannot possibly be cured by one remedy and inasmuch as the symptoms form part respectively of groups of different causations, covering the totality of all the symptoms present in the patient would be a useless and fruitless task. Hence it is that Rademacherian organ-testing helps me so much in my every-day practical clinical life; for, if I cure an organ with its *Appropriatum Paracelsi,* and certain symptoms go while others remain I am enabled slowly to unravel the most complex groups of symptoms and finally find a simile or even the simillimum of ·the ground-evil.

The adage *Naturam morborum ostendunt curationes* also comes in here as an auxiliary. With me it is an axiom to relieve uncomfortable or dangerous organ-states with simple organ-remedies as promptly as possible, leaving the more remote and deeper-going to be afterwards considered, and treated, if possible, with its pathological simillimum, or else ætiologically, say according to Hahnemann in his Coethen phase.

Carduus Mariæ IN ITS RELATION
WITH LIVER AND THE SKIN.

Perhaps it would be more correct
to think of the matter as twigs of
the same branch. Thus in my
small work on the Skin* I mention the seeming connection between the cutaneous surface of the
sternum and other internal affections, notably of the left lobe of the
liver therewith.

Subsequent experience has
taught me that although the
Carduus cures these cases very
promptly and indeed brilliantly,

---

* " Diseases of the Skin from the Organismic
Standpoint."—London, 1886.

still the cutaneous eruption is apt to recur.   In support of this connection; or, perhaps, it might be wiser to say concomitancy, I there give some *Carduus* cases thus:—

THE "STERNAL PATCH."·

One often meets with liver affections connected with cutaneous manifestations.

I would like particularly to refer to a patch of eruption on the skin covering the lower part of the sternum which I have several times found co-exist with heart disease and swelling of the left lobe of the liver.   In my case-takings I call it the "sternal patch."

I have four such cases in my mind at this moment, the first I will narrate is that of a mayor of a large town in the north:—He had a patch of brownish eruption on the sternal portion of thorax of the size of a woman's palm; with it were associated an enlarged liver and a cardiac affection evidenced by palpitation, systolic murmur, and general uneasiness. He came to town to see me at odd intervals for about two years, and was then discharged cured. He has passed under my observation since, but though his liver gives no trouble the same cannot be said of his skin, and he has moreover *pyorrhœa alveolaris.*

I treated him antipsorically and organopathically, the most notable benefit being derived from *Carduus mariæ* in five drop doses of the strong tincture given three times a day.

The second I remember was a Manchester merchant, with the same kind of cutaneous patch on the sternum, and very notable heart trouble with arcus senilis as a concomitant. Here the ease and comfort brought by the *Carduus mariæ* were very striking. Under date of January 31, 1883, I find in my case book these words of the enthusiastic patient—"It had a most marvellous effect, soon made me right; the patch went away

in a fortnight; had had it for years."

This gentlemen has remained under my care, calling upon me at odd times when in town, and during the past two years has had besides the strong tincture of *Carduus*, *Bellis perennis* 1, *Aurum Metallicum* 4, *Vanadium* 6, and *Acidum oxalicum* 3^x, and some other remedies, and I consider him vastly improved, and his life—speaking commercially—worth 40 per cent. more than previously.

The third case was that of a New York merchant, who suffered from liver and had come over to Europe to consult a physician, as he seemed to get no better from

6

the treatment of his New York advisers. I found his liver very much enlarged, and also the before-mentioned sternal patch of skin-disease. I gave him *Carduus* in like dose to the foregoing, and he came in a week declaring himself quite well. I advised him to re-main awhile under observation, to see if the cure proved permanent, but he hurried out of my room in great glee, and I never saw him again.

The fourth case in which I found the sternal patch and enlarged liver, giddiness, and palpitations of the heart was that of a London lawyer. Here the liver got well, and the heart too, together with

the giddiness, but it needed a course
of antipsoric treatment to finish
the cure of the patch of diseased
skin.   I might say the same of a
fifth case, an officer in the Royal
Navy, where this patch co-exists
with hypertrophied liver, and in
which the affair has a specific air
about it, probably inherited, and it
may be that when Sarcognomy is
better understood, and when the
relations of the various cutaneous
regions will be recognized as con-
stituting the very base of medical and medicinal diagnosis, this
sternal patch will be understood to
indicate "liver and heart."

But the following CASE CURED
BY *Carduus* is also instructive in

considering its relationship to skin and liver.

A city merchant, thirty years of age, unmarried, came to me in May, 1888, for windy dyspepsia, the probable ground-work of which proved to be an enlargement both of liver and spleen, and he had amongst other things very numerous sebaceous cysts strewn about his body, looking for all the world like the malva seeds (cases), children call cheeses.

At first I gave *Ceanothus Americanus*, believing it to be primarily a spleen affection, and then *Pulsatilla*, but they did no great good; when *Carduus*, given for a little over a month, brought the liver back to the normal and all the wee wens were gone.

The enlargement of the liver and the wens disappeared simultaneously, but the genuinely causal nature of both was neither hepatic nor cutaneous: That was scrofula. But as scrofula can only be treated in its manifestations, he who treats such manifestations successfully cures it. The general improvement under *Carduus* was most striking and lasting: patient got quite well and has since happily married.

E. Stahl speaks in his Dissertations most highly of *Carduus* in those inflammations of the chest which are accompanied by gall fevers, and it was from him that Rademacher first learned its use and never ceased to prize it, notably in blood spitting from liver and spleen engorgements. No remedy, he declares, in our whole drug store can compare to *Carduus* when there are stitches in the side with bloody expectoration. He recommends his readers to note well where the last trace of pain is felt as it dies away, as that is likely to be the primary seat of the real disease.

CASE OF JAUNDICE IN A NEW-BORN BABE CURED BY *Myrica Cerifera.*

An able accoucheur attended a lady who bore a jaundiced babe; said he, "I cannot give that wee thing any medicine, so you had better send for your homœopath (meaning me), as he can give some of his 'pips'!" This was done and pilules of *Myrica cerifera* 3[×] (crushed into a powder and rubbed on the baby's tongue) rapidly cured him, and he at once began to put on flesh, and has thriven ever since. Before taking the *Myrica* he was very weedy, thin, and leathery-looking.

Myrica cerifera is one of the

very valuable additions to our *materia medica* that have come to us from America. I have often used it in liver disease, notably in bad cases of jaundice, with striking success; it produces jaundice in the healthy pathogenetically, and is very searching in its action. It was the great American Samuel Thomson, the botanic practitioner, who brought it into notice. A pale green wax is obtained from its berries, and hence it is called *ceriferus*, or wax-bearing. Its powdered bark was Thomson's "canker powder," and he advised it in all discharges from the mucous surfaces, especially in leucorrhœa, dysentery, and nasal catarrh.

Dr. Leland Walker's proving, as given in "Hale's New Remedies," shews an accurate picture of severe catarrhal jaundice; we are, therefore, on indisputably scientific ground when we prescribe *Myrica* for catarrhal jaundice. No wonder that the old American botanists practised with so much success. That Thomson was a close and accurate observer may be seen from the fact that he commends it to "disengage the thick viscid secretions of the mucous membrane," for we find Walker's pathogenetic Myrica-catarrh was of the same viscid quality; he says: "throat and nasal organs filled with an offensive *tenacious* mucus."

LEPTANDRA VIRGINICA

Is another valuable contribution from America, effecting the liver, mucous membrane, lungs, and pleura. Roughly, it is the mercury of the eclectics. It has never been a favorite of mine, simply because I have not needed it, inasmuch as it closely resembles *Chelidonium* in its effects. I once saw Dr. Reginald Jones, of Birkenhead, make a brilliant cure of a severe case of right-sided pneumonia with it—its prompt, decisive, curative action was unmistakeable.

In the lazy livers of city men, I have used *Leptandrin* 3 in six-grain doses with great satisfaction to the patients.

SANGUINARIA CANADENSIS is, in truth, a liver medicine, but not primarily or principally so, and is too great a remedy to be mentioned only in passing.

PODOPHYLLUM PELTATUM is a great liver remedy, and has been greatly abused. Its use in "torpid liver" is not good practice, and has done much harm Its true scientific homœopathic use is in diarrhœa from overflowing bile, with much irritation, and even inflammation of the gut. It once stood me in good stead in a case of diarrhœa that threatened to end fatally—at any rate the allopathic family adviser had informed the lady's husband that he considered the patient would not recover, as nothing would check the diarrhœa, and the lady was seemingly sinking. I was telegraphed for and had to travel nearly 200 miles. On arriving, the family physician, although he had given the patient up as past recovery, declined to meet me because of my homœopathic creed, and this although he professed to be a friend of the family, and only lived two doors off. The stools were foul smelling, hot, bilious, excoriating, and passed out of the anus in a constant dribble. The patient had become too weak to be raised or even adequately helped, and things had to be just left. I studied the case a short time, and finally decided upon *Podophyllum* 6. The next evening patient was convalescent, and I returned to town. The cure was complete and permanent. When the family physician had heard of my departure, he returned and very kindly watched the case for me, still giving my remedy. "Why," said he, "Podophyllum is one of our allopathic medicines it is not a homœopathic medicine at all; they have stolen it from us."

The poor ignoramus still knows not that the *use* of the remedy, *i. e.*, the principle on which it is used, is the point at issue.

It might be asked, why would this dapper medico not meet the writer over a supposedly dying patient, and would yet accept the more humble position of merely watching the case and giving my remedy after I had departed?

It was thus: He and another doctor in the place each considered himself the first man there; and if his rival had heard that he had met a homœopathic practitioner in proper consultation, he would have been denounced for unprofessional conduct, and his status lowered in the eyes of dear Mrs. and Dr. Grundy. He declared to the family that he personally should have been de-

lighted to have met me, but that
he had to consider his own position.

Such is medical life here in
England to-day. Still, for all that,
Podophyllum 6, humanly speaking,
saved the lady's life; and I, having
done my duty, have therein my
reward, and I thank God for the
privilege.

In the debility from jaundice
I have found *Picric acid* very
helpful. I have commonly used it
in the third dilution.

I have found the *Brassica
murialis*, which Dr. Heath tells
me should be called *Diplotaxis*
7

tenuifolia, of good service in the lazy livers of relaxing climates, when patients feel as if they could scarcely crawl about from sheer goneness. It is homœopathic to such, as I know from a fragmentary proving made by myself in 1874.

GALLSTONES.

In the treatment of gallstones we have to consider the attacks of gall colic and the treatment of the stones themselves when they lie in the gall bladder giving no one any trouble. I have treated gallstones and gallstone colic a good many times with hepatics of various

kinds, and have found myself best
in the painful attacks with *Hydrastis Canadensis*, originally given
from a suggestion of Dr. Henry
Thomas. A great many remedies
stand in good repute for the treatment of this almost unique complaint. I have used as much
as ten-drop doses of the strong
tincture of *Hydrastis*, given every
half-hour in very warm water, and
known it to succeed in a few hours
after everything had failed. In
one case the patient had· lain for
40 hours in terrible agony, un-
relieved by any known thing. It
is odd that people who have been
taking *Hydrastis*, not infrequently
think they have been taking

7

Opium. After the attack of pain
is over, it is best to set about
curing the liver itself by a long
course of homœopathically-indica-
ted remedies, whose names are
legion; for it must be manifest
that gallstones are a secondary
affection, due to a previous condition either of the liver or of the
gall, or of the gall-bladder, or of
the linings of the ducts. In some
cases I have thought the whole
state had started originally in
catarrhal jaundice.

My own procedure I will exemplify by narrating a case in
point at some length.

CASE OF GALLSTONES AND ORGANIC DISEASE OF LIVER.

A lady of fifty years of age came under my observation early in the year 1888 with a very muddy complexion, subicteric whites of the eyes. She suffered very much from acidity and also from vomiting.

She told me she had been a sufferer from her liver for many years; severe bilious headaches and dyspepsia. She had been mercurialized for her liver till all her teeth fell out, and now her digestion had given in almost completely, and she had become so thin that her appearance was quite cachectic. She had got so frightened of anything bringing on her attacks of gall colic that she avoided almost every article of food.

Owing to her great emaciation and trim build I was able to make the diagnosis of gallstones from actually feeling them, a thing I am very rarely able to do myself. The region of the gall-bladder was, however, so tender that a very little feeling with my hands was as much as she could bear. I treated her for close upon two years, and then she was a plump, bonny woman, enjoying her life and dining out with her friends. Her skin had become comparatively healthy looking, though not as clear as a healthy English lady's generally is.

I chose the remedies on homœopathic indications, and here and there as Rademacher would have done; and, when I the last few times examined the region of the gall-bladder, I entirely failed to find any stones.

She had the following remedies seriatim, *Ignatio amara* 1×, *Chelidonium* 1× and *Φ*, *Nux vomica* 1×, *Cholesterine* 3×, *Hydrastis Can. Φ*, *Thuja occ.* 30, *Sanguinaria Can. Φ*, *Carduus mariæ Φ*, and *Bilirubin.* 5. All these remedies did their portion of the good, and were given as they were indicated.

I have rarely seen a more satisfactory cure of a difficult, almost desperate, chronic case, and quite as rarely had a patient, with a worse family history. Which remedy cured the patient? All of them.

There is a *Carduus* case that should have come in earlier on, but I had mislaid the MS., and as it is short I will add it here, and principally because it neatly exemplifies the *Carduus* action. Five years have elapsed since the patient was cured, and there has been no return of any of the symptoms, and he has continued otherwise in uninterruptedly good health.

HYPERTROPHY OF LEFT LOBE OF THE LIVER; SLIGHT HYPERTROPHY OF THE HEART; STERNAL PATCH.

On January 27th, 1885, a young gentleman, twenty-one years of age, and who had long been ailing of no one seemed to know what, was sent by his father to me " to be thoroughly overhauled and put right." The overhauling disclosed slight enlargement of the heart, considerable enlargement of the left lobe of the liver, and a very prominent sternal patch. Patient complained of suffering a good deal from giddiness.

℞ *Carduus mariæ* φ, five drops in water night and morning.

He was discharged permanently cured in six months. During a considerable portion of the time he was taking the *Carduus*, which quite set heart and liver right, but the sternal patch I had to cure nosodically, of which . . . *une autre fois.* I often see members of this gentleman's family, including his parents, and know, as I said just now, that he has continued well ever since.

We will now return to gall-stones.

An elderly lady came under my observation early in the summer

of 1888, for gallstones, character-
ized by frequent recurrent attacks
of jaundice, colic, and vomiting,
with the usual agonizing pains.
She was under me a good many
month—about eighteen, if I remember rightly—and then discontinued her treatment, and has
since continued well. I strongly
urged her to go on longer, lest
there should still be present the
remains of the old colic-causing
stones, but to no avail Why
should I continue taking medicines
when I am well?

She had in succession (and
several repeatedly), *Kali bichromi-
cum*, *Carduus mariæ*, *Hydrastis
Canadensis*, *Prunus Virginiana*,

Cholesterine, iodoformum, and finally *Ferrum picricum* 3^×. The last
named medicine does capital service in bilious debility.

CASE OF COLIC FROM GALLSTONES.

A middle-aged gentleman
brought his wife to me three
years since to be treated for gallstones, and the usual attacks of
colic with vomiting, that came on
at odd intervals, from known and
unknown causes. Patient had
been long under their own doctor
in the country, but to no good
purpose; in fact, a chronic pain in
the right side had been superadded
to the before-mentioned colic at-

tacks, and patient had lost flesh a good deal. She paid me visits once a month for many months, until she was quite well and in a thoroughly thriving condition.

However, I told the husband that I did not think the biliary calculi were really entirely gone, and that I thought it would be wise to continue with the use of gentle gall-medicines till we had sounder ground for believing that there would be no further relapses.

But patient seemed and looked in such capital health that there really seemed, from their standpoint, no reason for continuing my treatment, so my warning was not regarded.

The remedies that helped so brilliantly in this case were *Hydrastis*, *Carduus*, *Chelidonium* and *Berberis*, and two or three others which I have not noted.

It must be fully a year since saw any of the family, but this morning I was prescribing for her brother-in-law, who told me that she is now lying in the country very ill with gallstones, and her attending physicians consider her case hopeless. So all experience goes to show that the after-treatment of gallstones should be carried on for a very long time, so as to get rid of the disease altogether. Long delay at the printers' enables me to add that after having been thus given up, this lady again placed herself under my care, and has at last completely recovered her health, *Euonymin* and *Thlaspi bursa pastoris* φ having helped most.

How the biliary calculi are dissolved I am unable to say; that they *are* eventually really and truly got rid of by dissolution I infer from the fact that the sufferers get well and remain so.

It might be asked: What is your indication for *Bursa pastoris* in Gallstones?

Answer: When the *original* liver-ailing *started* primarily from the womb. I will refer to this again.

Chronic Biliousness and Emaciation Cured by *Chelidonium.*

A strumous gentleman, about thirty years of age, came over from Ireland to consult me with regard to loss of flesh, dyspepsia, and biliousness. He was over six feet in height, and only weighed ten stone. Hair reddish; thorax flat; pronounced venous zig-zag; digestion very weak; poor appetite; a brownish rash across the epigastrium; cannot digest vegetables.

The state of the liver led me to prescribe *Chelidonium* 1; five drops in water night and morning.

Under this prescription (with the same diet, occupation, and place of abode as previously), he increased five pounds in weight in thirty-two days. In six months he had reached 10-stone 12 lbs. in weight, and he long after reported to me that he had "remained in very good health, indeed." Besides being for some months under the influence of *Chelidonium*, he had inter-currently also *Badiaga* 3$^\times$ and *Psorinum* 30, each during one month.

The state of the skin caused me to interpose *Psorinum*, and some symptoms of indigestion led me to give the *Badiaga*.

8

But the strikingly great amelioration set in first under the sole
influence of the *Chelidonium*, but
this remedy did not extend its
influence far enough or wide
enough, and hence it had to be
supplemented by the other two,
but with the spheres of action of
them we are here not concerned.

ENLARGEMENT OF LIVER, PRODUCING SHORTNESS OF BREATH AND PALPITATION, CURED BY *Chelidonium majus* $3^\times$.

Some years since a retired merchant, sixty-eight years of age,
consulted me for a supposed affection of his heart.. He complained

of obesity, fulness in the stomach,
violent perspirations on moving
about—so much so that he was in
the habit of changing shirts during
the forenoon already; feels puffy
on going up a hill; loses his breath
from the stomach on the least hurry.
Has a fresh healthy look.   No arcus senilis.   Is very active, and
takes a good deal of exercise.

After taking twenty drops of
Chelidonium maj. 3× per diem for a
few weeks I noted, at his dictation:
" The puffiness is much better; I
can walk with greater ease; I feel as
if something were gone from me."
That is to say, his swelled liver
had gone down and there was more
playroom for his lungs and heart.

He weighed 15-stone 9 lbs., and under the action of *Chelidonium* this came down to 15-stone 6 lbs.

He afterwards had *Chelidonium* 1, and also *Euonymin* $3^{\times}$, and after 15 months' treatment he had gone down one stone in weight, and was able to go up hill and upstairs with comfort.

I saw him a year ago for neuralgia, when *Silicea* 200 was followed by the disappearance of the neuralgia.

CASE OF GALL COLIC CURED BY *Myrica Cerifera* 3×. .

In the year 1889 a lady of some 30 odd years of age came to consult me for her liver. She seemed healthy and bright, but severe pains in her right side, pyrosis, and certain brown patches on her skin clearly implicated the liver. Patient took for a month *Chelidonium* φ with distinct benefit. She afterwards had *Ignatia amara* 1 and subsequently *Hydrastis Can.* φ, and both with some considerable benefit.

She came then to town to see me, when I again failed to find anything to account for her dyspepsia, though the pain I could trace clearly to the gall-bladder.

After taking *Myrica cerif.* 3$^{\times}$, five drops in a table-spoonful of water, for some weeks, I received a very grateful letter from her, in which she says: "That medicine has done me a great deal of good; I have lost all pain in my side, and have had only one headache, and no indigestion, and I walk six miles a day."

What the exact state of the gall-ducts was of course I could not tell; I could not feel any calculi; none had ever been passed, she thought.

Although *Chelidonium* and *Hydrastis* both did much good, it was the *Myrica* that really hit the mark curatively.

When a patient gets the *right* organ-remedy it is often really astonishing how their feeling of *bien-être* is augmented: they not only *become well*, they very emphatically *feel it;* they are, as it were aggressively well.

Of course, a good complexion means health, more or less, but the liver is very specially involved in producing a clean skin and clear complexion; and I propose by-and-bye to dilate upon this point

somewhat, as I consider it impor
tant.*

CASE OF TAWNINESS OF SKIN,
BRONCHIAL CATARRH,
AND COUGH.

The tawny skin is met with in
greatest perfection in those who
have lived in hot countries; and
where this dirty-looking dinginess
of the skin is not from constitutional disease, or inherited from
phthisically-disposed parents* it is
quite amenable to treatment. The
tawny discoloration can be more or
less removed. This tawniness I re-

---

*See, on this subject, my "Five Years' Ex-
perience in the New Cure of Consumption."

gard as chronic subicterism, and, indeed, the anti-icterics cure such cases beautifully. They generally take a good deal of time to be really and permanently cured, and a whole series of such remedies have to be brought into play in succession, one after the other, together with here and there an inter-current nosode; but at times they will mend quickly from one or two remedies only.

Thus at the beginning of the current year a city merchant, fifty-five years of age, came to consult me for a cough, with a bronchial catarrh. The tawniness of his skin was very marked, and this he attributed to a twenty years' residence in Africa. The cough was habitual, and worse in the evening. There are a good many crescentic cutaneous efflorescences on his chest.

Two months of *Hydrastis Canadensis* Φ.

He took altogether just an ounce, in small material doses. Cured the cough; reduced the catarrh of the bronchial lining to a minimum; and very materially lessened the tawniness of his skin; many of his friends remarking upon the very striking improvement in his seemingly dirty complexion. I should have followed up with some three or four other anti-icterics, but the gentleman considered he was well enough, and would not come any more, even "please his wife."

THE COMPLEXION OF THE SKIN IN RELATION TO LIVER AFFECTIONS.

That the complexion is more or less modified in certain affections of the liver is pretty patent to all the world, and the least observant readily remarks that "So-and-so's liver cannot be right." Nevertheless, when people's skins are in an unhealthy state they commonly treat the skin, or go to a skin doctor who is pretty sure to regard his specialty as the first, and treats the skin, generally *d'en face*, with washes and ointments and the like.

I have tried to combat this view in my "Diseases of the Skin from the Organismic Standpoint," but, I am afraid, with too little success.

The skin gets its life from within; it is fed from within from the blood, and it is from within that a good complexion must be obtained. One cannot make an unhealthy skin healthy by any washes or ointments whatsoever.

I have preached this doctrine before and oft, but few will listen, and hence I am going to preach it again, so that I may at least be able to say *dixi et animam meam salvavi.*

Take a person whose skin is jaundiced. Does anyone propose to wash the yellow skin white?

And if not, why not? It were almost as rational as to try to get a good complexion from any powders and washes whatsoever, and yet the deluded apply such things daily in faith believing.

LARGE VARICOSE VEIN; ENLARGEMENT OF LIVER.

It might be wondered at, that I should give a case of varicosis in a work devoted to the main diseases of the liver, but, as a matter of fact, the case is so unique that I add it here lest it be lost, and because I hardly know where it would fit in better.

At the beginning of 1889, a young lady was brought to me by her mother for a large varicose vein running from her right shoulder, over the right clavicle, and across the upper half of the right side of the chest. It varied in size somewhat, and at its largest was about the size of an ordinary quill.

Being great society people this vein cast quite a shadow over their lives, it being "quite impossible, you know, to dress."

One sees the oddest things in the way of varicose veins in the lower half of the body, but not very often in the upper, as gravitation is enough to empty them when they are higher up.

All kinds of treatment had been applied, or applied to, and quite lately the vein had been treated by that wonderful cure-nothing—electricity.

I reasoned thus: Veins that dilate in that manner, steadily, slowly, increasingly, must do so from an obstruction in their progression heartwards, just as the little rivulets higher up the stream must fill up when the stream is dammed up lower down.

From a rather careful physical survey of the parts involved, I found the liver very large—indeed huge, which was probably accounted for by the fact that patient had thrice had ague, or else three attacks of the same. Her skin was dirty dingy-looking, and the portion covering the lower end of the breast bone studded with wee flat warts, and the degree of anæmia was considerable. Moreover, she had a disagreeable cough, and her sleep was not good.

An ounce of *Chelidonium* φ, spread over eleven weeks, restored the liver to its normal size, and the varicosis had almost entirely disappeared, so that patient had again taken to evening dress—respectively, undress. Her skin at the same time became clearer, and her blood of evidently better quality.

CASE OF GALLSTONES.

The wife of a well-known clergyman came under my observation on the 12th of June, 1889, for gallstones. Competent medical men had attended her in these attacks, and had diagnosed gallstones. Patient had turned fifty, and is the mother of many children. Her attacks began with sharp agonizing pains. in the pit of the stomach, extending to the arms, and with

9

them severe vomiting; her breath is very short; her bowels are costive, and she is a martyr to flatulent dyspepsia.

Being a rich woman, she had sought the best advice in London, but to no avail. Her physicians had stated that nothing more could be done. Her lower extremities had begun to swell, and this, coupled with a loss of flesh, dyspnœa, and a very darkly icteric coloration of the skin, seemed to corroborate the given prognosis, and the more so as patient's able physicians had long tried their best with such remedies as are current in the orthodox school of medicine.

But knowing well their poverty in remedies, and in knowledge of remedies, I set about treating this lady precisely as if she had never had any medical treatment at all.

Thirteen months later, while I am actually writing these notes, she is plump, healthy looking, and touring with her husband in Scotland, and she has had no pains at all for just eleven months. Friends who have not seen her for some time barely able to recognize her because of her changed appearance.

Her remedies were *Hydrastis Canadensis, Bryonia alba , Thuja occident., Helonium, Strophanthus,* and intercurrently, for far-reaching

9

constitutional effects, two common nosodes in high dilutions.

The change in this lady's dis-. position is rather remarkable, as from being dull, taciturn, unengaging, and almost socially uncivil, she has become bright, affable and chatty. The fact is, our brightness and chatty sunniness in our social life do verily depend much upon the liver.

Cholesterinum IN TUMOURS OF LIVER.

This is obtained from gall; I believe from that of the bullock. I learned its use of the late Dr. Ameke, of Berlin, author of the

"History of Homœopathy," translated into English by (alas, also the *late*) Dr. Alfred Drysdale, sometime of Cannes.

Ameke claimed to have derived much advantage from its use in *cancer of the liver*. This is a weighty statement, and is *true*. I believe I have twice cured cancer of the liver with it; and in obstinate hepatic engorgements that, by reason of their obstinacy, make one thing interrogatively of cancer, the effects of *Cholesterine* are very satisfactory; at times even striking.

I commonly use the $3^\times$ trit. in six-grain doses three times a day, but this will here and there act very violently, and when this happened I have found the third centesimal trituration effective.

Sometimes one meets with cases in which there appears to be a semi-malignant affection, involving the left lobe of the liver, and what lies between it and the pylorus and the pancreas, and here *Cholesterine* $3^\times$ and *Iodoformum* $3^\times$, in four-hourly alternation, have several times rendered me sound service.

I may relate one such. Summoned 60 miles into the country late one afternoon, to a supposedly dying lady of 60 odd years of age, I found her icteric, vomiting, bathed in cold perspiration, very thin, *débile;* the pulse small and weak, and patient seemingly almost moribund. Nothing would stay on the stomach. The seat of the affection was the left lobe of the liver, extending to the left and towards the navel. That there were gallstones is probable, but, quite *outside* of the acute attack, there was a chronic affection of some kind in the region just named, evidenced by swelling and tenderness.

Kali bich. 5 relieved; *Cholesterine* 3× and *Iodof.* 3× cured in a month, and, the case being of long standing, the cure converted several families to the contemned pathy of Samuel Hahnemann.

But, allowing for all doubtfulness and vagueness in what I here relate, *Cholesterine* is my sheet-anchor in organic liver disease in which the commoner hepatics— *Chelid.,Carduus,Myrica,Kali bich.,* *Merc.,* and *Diplotaxis tenuifolia* have failed.

I do not think that *Chlosterine* has any influence upon the "disposition" to cancer, but it acts by reason of its elective affinity for the seat of the disease; it effects therefore not a cure in the Hunternian sense, inasmuch as it only gets rid of the product of the disease, but that is something, as there is then a temporary cure, which under favorable circum-

stances may become permanent
proof of which permanence of curative results I will presently ad-
duce. In this case the cure has
proved to be permanent, as now
(two years since the lady is in
capital health, and on a visit to
her daughter in the North of
England.

CURING THE INCURABLE—THE INSOLENCE OF IGNORANCE.

" Le cancer est incurable parcèqu' on ne le guérit pas ordinairement; on ne peut le guérir puisqu 'il est incurable, donc quand on le guérit c'est qu'il n' existait pas."—*Duparcque*.

The saying of Duparcque which stands at the head of this, pithily puts the whole question; the thing has not changed, *c'est alors comme alors*.

This I will dwell upon very briefly now, and at the same time bear the very highest testimony to the virtues of *Cholesterine* in cancer of the liver.

On January 30th, 1889, an American gentleman, confessing to sixty-five years of age, and on a visit to his daughter, married to an English clergyman in the north, was accompanied to my rooms by the said daughter, so ill was he that had I thereafter heard of his immediate demise I should have been not in the very least astonished.

The note taken at the time stands thus in my case book under the above date . . . . Thin, weak, débile; yellow conjunctivæ, insomnia : very nervous and ap-

prehensive. Been treated for enlarged liver and had lots of calomel
and chloral. His skin is tawny,
cachectic. There is a swelling of
the liver or of the pancreas—probably malignant disease of the left
lobe of the liver. Always suffered
from dyspepsia. Been a great
ocean traveler. "I am very fond
of salt, and eat a great deal." Is
a practical teetotaler. Bones of
the fingers very knobby He is
a spring-and-fall ailer. Has lost
a stone weight since November.
Never been ill but ailing, and has
taken much medicine: bromides
and chloral, urethran. Very chilly.
He is very ill. Urine normal. Has
had ague, ond been twice vaccinated.

I ordered him six grains of the third decimal trituration of *Cholesternium* every four hours, and requested him to call in a few days. The married daughter demanded my candid opinion, and I said it was, in my judgment, cancer of the liver, when she informed me that that was the unanimous opinion of all their medical advisers the most trusted of whom were quite sure the lethal end was not far off.

That would also have been my opinion had I not seen *Cholesterine* bring back hope in several desperate cases of cancer of the liver. I therefore felt warranted in stating that I thought our remedies carefully and persistently applied might yet cure him. In a few days patient returned to me in company with his daughter, and I hardly like to say what the change was, so great was the amelioration. He looked vastly improved and walked firmly, and indeed already considered himself on the high road to recovery, almost wondering what all the fuss had been about.

When Mr. D. R. had retired, his daughter very anxiously said, "What do you think, now?" I said I had not altered my opinion; and that the improvement was due to the remedy and not natural recovery, and that the said improvement would have to be followed up with close scientific treatment which might, and indeed most likely would, result in a positive and direct art-cure. I also tried to explain that we had begun successfully and rapidly to deal with the product of the disease, and that done we could proceed to deal with the disposition thereto. I ordered patient to go on another few days with the prescription which I had given to him at first (*Cholest.*,) and then to report himself to me.

In about half an hour thereafter the daughter returned with her husband, and the latter almost flew at me in very rage. "What," said he, "do you mean to tell me that

my wife's father has cancer?"
"Yes." "And that you are going
to cure him?" "Yes. I think I
shall, but I am not sure." Here-
upon he raised his voice somewhat
and repeated his questions so offen-
sively that I turned away from
him and he left. I have never seen
or heard of any of them since; nor
have I ever since seen the wife's
sister, Lady ——, whom I cured in
1886 of a thickening of the Cardia,
but Lady ——'s cure was a truly
Hunterian one, and she has been
quite well for long. I have been
so often amazed at the insolence of
ignorance that I not infrequently
find it hard to bear with equanimity.
Thus here I was positively in-

sulted, essentially because I knew more on a given point than certain others, viz., that *Cholesterine* will at any rate curatively modify some cases that seem to be hepatic carcinosis.

Still, I thank God and take comfort . . . they know not what they do.

People who are sick of some chronic disease and are given over to their fate by those who ought at least to have the courage of hopefulness, find not infrequently their greatest enemies in their nearest relations, who resent efforts at cure. These Job's comforters seem to regard determined efforts to cure their friends as personal insults.

This phenomenon I have observed so often that I have wondered what the explanation thereof might be: in ultimate analysis it would seem to be human vanity. _They_ have pronounced the case hopeless, and therefore it is so and not otherwise.

Ubi morbus ibi remedium.

This idea is very old, and clings to mankind with wonderful tenaciousness. On this is founded Ameke's conception which, had he been spared would, I think, have resulted at least in the discovery of notable remedies for which clinical experience would subsequently have afforded fixed indications.

TUMOUR OF LIVER OF GREAT SIZE CURED BY *Cholesterinum.*

A country squire nearing seventy years of age came under my observation in the early part of 1889 for a very large tumour clearly connected with the left lobe of the liver. Patient was so ill that he reached town with difficulty, and became so weak that it was impossible for him to return.

Orthodoxy well represented had given him up; and his profound adynamia and cachectic look warranted me in stating that I had but small hope. But he was a plucky

10

fellow—a type of the British aristocrat (born to govern and fit therefor: because living out of doors and *not* reading books— Beaconsfield) and he was willing to obey to the letter.

I advised him to go to the Grand Hotel and quarter himself in the sunny front high up out of the dirt and din, and there abide. He did so, and a very pleasant abode that is: the sun streaming in; the quiet; and yet the outlook upon the seething mass below, which keeps from stagnation.

A homœopath for half a century he had boundless faith in *Nux vomica*, but I told him that

I was sure *Nux* would not cure him, and as this visibly depressed him, I said I would give him my medicine, but in alternation with it he should have his *Nux*. Hence this was given in alternation with *Cholesterine.* The tumour slowly disappeared, the liver went down to the state it had been in for forty years, *i. e.* the left lobe somewhat bulging, and patient returned to his country seat in about two months, and ever since he is not, as a rule, conscious of possessing a liver at all, though once in a way he feels a little uneasy in the hepatic region. This I know, as patient has long been worried with vesical catarrh, and for this I am now treating him, keeping all the time a certain amount of attention directed to the hepatic region in case of any further explosion; for I do not imagine that the cure thus far is a truly Hunterian one.

True, the tumour is gone and may never recur, and the gentleman has a very healthy look; but, after all, the tumour is not itself the disease, but the disease-product.

I would not be understood to maintain that a tumour which thus goes from drug action on the *ubi morbus ibi remedium* idea must necessarily recur, but that it may But I will continue on this same subject in my next chapter.

At the time of going to press this gentleman continues well.

AMEKEAN TREATMENT OF HEPA-
TIC TUMOURS; HEPTIC CANCER.

About five years ago, a gentleman of 67 or thereabouts came
under my observation for a swelling under the right ribs that competent authorities had diagnosed
as of a cancerous nature. It had
come a good many months subsequent to an accident: a cab wheel
having gone over the body at the
part mentioned. He had been
under a good West-end homœopathic physician who had agreed,
after a close examination, to the
diagnosis, and declared positively
to the gentleman's wife that he
had no hope whatever of curing

the case, and he thought it his duty to say so.

The whole thing was quite cured with the remedies in about a year; the most striking, palpable result being observed after the use of *Cholesterine* in different dilutions, though numerous remedies were needed as well, notably *Carduus mariæ* φ, *Chelidonium majus* φ, *Myrica cerifera* 3ˣ, *Iodium* 1, *Kali bich.* 5, and *Nat. mur.* 6 trit.

Five years have elapsed and there has been no recurrence of tumour, and during the whole of the five years the gentleman has only been away from his business for three weeks and that was to go to the seaside last August.

A few days since I saw his wife on her own account, when she reported him "quite well."

This certainly looks like a Hunterian cure. I can now report on another and very similar case, as follows:—

ANOTHER *Cholesterinum* CASE.

Nearly six years ago, indeed a little longer, as it was early in the year 1876, I was required to treat a liver case almost exactly like the foregoing one. But patient was not much over fifty years of age then, and it arose primarily, it was thought, from adhesive peritonitis

of long before. Eor years this gentlemen, a county man, had felt the
jolting in a carriage at first uncomfortable, and latterly so painful
that he had got into the habit of
holding his hand against the
swelled part to support it and prevent its feeling the effects of the
shaking.

With the sole addition of *Me-
dorrh. C.* the treatment was as in
the last case, and of about the same
duration, viz., about a year, and
with an equally satisfactory result:
he got well, and has remained well
to date, working very hard almost
all the time. This I know, as he
has come about four times a year
to be assured that his old enemy

had been, not merely scotched, but killed.

In this case I myself originally gave a bad prognosis to the gentleman's wife, and it was the *Cholesterine* that brought life and hope into the matter. It is very difficult to cure a tumid mass of any kind with one remedy: one needs Organopathy, Homœopathy, Amekeanism, and empiricism, together with theories no end, if the full extent of the possible is to be attained.

In my judgment the full range of the art-cure of disease by remedies used on scientific lines starts from the due recognition of the primary seat of the disease, and of the remedies that electively affect such primary seat. This, I take it, is the homœopathic specificity of seat. Experience teaches me that if we are to avoid false issues in treatment we must *start* with diagnosing, if possible, *where* the malady is primarily located. At any rate, I find this the *shortest* way to curing. If this be neglected we not infrequently cover and cure the symptoms, leaving the malady itself more or less untouched.

No doubt—and on this I lay some stress—when the symptoms are scientifically (*i. e.* homœopathically) covered and cured, the disease causing the symptoms is at the same time often radically cured also; but also, and not seldom, the symptoms are got rid of, but the disease remains.

It has been urged that any untrained person can treat homœo-pathically by mechanically covering the symptoms ; and no doubt, this is, to some extent, true. But such cures are not worth much; they do not reach very far, and are only of practical value when the malady and the symptoms are convertible terms. The simillimum of the symptoms may, *or may not* be the simillimum of the malady ; if of latter, we have an ideal therapy beyond which there is nought to be desired ; if of the symptoms only, we are apt to keep on curing our patients till they die.

If homœopathy is to go on advancing we must face the question of *getting behind the symptoms*, so that we may not only treat the symptoms homœopathically, but also the malady in its essence. In other words, it will not suffice to find the simillimum of the symptoms, but that being found, it will be needful to put this pertinent question : Is this symptomatic simillimum also homœopathic to the anatomical essence of the malady itself ?

In the simple and well-defined forms of disease affecting an isolated organ, Paracelsic homœopathy or organopathy is a very valuable guide to cure, and helps to define the disease and to fix its cure with the *pathalogic simile.*

This results from a recognition that certain organs of the body are, as it were, organisms within the organism; minor systems within the general system. They have special individualism, both as to their functions and as to their diseases. Such an organ is the liver. It can be made ill by the organism, but, in its turn, it can make the organism ill. They act and re-act upon one another. Neither can exist without the other.

Certain drugs have been discovered by man, almost in all places

and at all times, that have an
elective affinity for these organs,
and these drugs have some of them
received names indicative of their
action, hence we have head medicines, spleen medicines, liver medicines.

This small volume is intended
to shew that the greater or more
common Diseases of the Liver can,
for the most part, be readily cured
by hepatics or liver medicines.

Inasmuch as a large number of
hepatics are well-known to us, our
chief difficulty lies in finding out
which remedy will cure a *given case*.
How far I have succeeded in over-
coming this difficulty is shewn in

these pages, and where I fail,
others, beginning where I leave
off, may succeed.

The cure of organ-diseases by
organ-remedies is often called organopathy, and this it was that
very largely constituted the practice of Paracelsus, and for which
he was hounded to death. His
success was so great that envy and
hatred arose and fiercely attacked
him. There can be no doubt that
Paracelsus was foully murdered by
the hired servants of his fellow-
practitioners; and oh! the number
of medical tomtits that have thrown
dirt on his memory all through the
after-living generations!

For all that, his great genius

11

flames still bright above the horizon, lighting up the life-paths of such as have the power to see. It supplies light, but not eyes.

I would remind those homœopathic practitioners who throw their little handfuls of dirt at Paracelsus that it was he—Paracelsus—who planted the acorn from which the mighty oak of homœopathy has grown.

It was just as impossible for Paracelsus to work out a homœopathic equation on the purely scientific ground of drug physiology or provings as did Hahnemann, as it was impossible for the farmers in the time of Hahnemann to use the steam plough *i. e.* it was not there to be used.

I have long mainted that organopathy is elementary homœopathy —that in the very nature of things, homœopathy necessarily includes organopathy.

Paracelsus was an organopath, being the founder of organopathy. I think it most likely that he picked up its elements and elementary principles on his travels, applied them in practice, and having made cures that have rarely been equalled, he systematized it. Personally I acknowledge my great indebtedness to Paracelsus, (largely through Rademacher) with all gratitude. I am constantly and in-

11'

cre- ingly impressed with the importance of ascertaining the exact *primary* seat of any localised malady, and I have been driven to this by certain of my failures in purely symptomatic treatment. To really and radically heal of disease, one must often dig down and find out where the *fons et origo mali* is, and to this end Paracelsic organ-testing is of the very greatest service; indeed it often leads to the most important clinical discovery. And what may the *most* important clinical discovery be? That which *nec dextrosum, nec sinistrosum* leads straight to the goal of every true physician—mastery over disease, *i. e.*, its direct art-cure.

CASE OF GALLSTONES AND ASTHMA.

It must be nearly ten years ago that a widow lady from abroad came to consult me for asthma and biliary calculi: and I will relate her case, not only because it is apposite as a cure of a liver affection, but because the lady has been more or less within my professional ken ever since, and at this present time she is in very good health, and for long has had neither Asthma nor Gallstone attacks.

Another point of interest for me lies in the fact that four well-known homœopathic physicians had treated the case during over three years with only indifferent success. They treated the symptoms without any physical diagnosis, and after having prescribed for the symptoms and temporarily cured many of them, the patient remained pretty much where she was before. Had they gone into the case they would have found that the bronchial asthma, retching and vomiting had their *point de départ* in the gall bladder.

No doubt this had again its origin in the constitutional crasis of the individual, and hence I began the treatment with very infrequent doses of *Psoricum* 30. This much lessened the pain in the right side, and it greatly relieved the cough. Then during about five weeks patient was under the influence of *Chelidonium* 1, and pain and cough quite disappeared.

In a fortnight the pain starting from the gall bladder returned, and was accompanied with much retching. Patient was of opinion that the side pain had originally come from taking such quantities of phosphorus for her cough years ago. At any rate, she affirmed that she never felt pain in this region before.

There is no return of asthma since she left off the *Chelidonium*.

I next prescribed *Terebinthina*

$3^\times$, four drops in water three times a day. The *Tereb.* rather upset her at first, and then she got better.

After this an attack of gall colic came on from exertion.

The duskiness of the skin, and the big brown patches on the forehead, led me to give *Nux.* It did much good, and under its influence patient's skin became lighter and cleaner. Then followed *Thuja* 30, and subsequently at odd intervals, according to the symptoms, *Mercurius vivus, Antimon. tart.* 3, *Pulsatilla* $3^\times$, *Cholesterine* 2, *Ipec., Alnus rub., Nat. Sul.* 6, and *Calc. carb.* 30.

But these were mostly for the

gallstones, as there had never been any return of the asthma after the *Psoricum* followed by the *Cheli-donium*, and that is more than nine years ago.

This I consider the more re-markable, as both her own mother and her own son had asthma; and an asthmatic lady, daughter and mother of individuals similarly afflicted, would hardly have a tran-sitory or spurious kind of asthma.

RADEMACHER'S HEPATIC

Rademacher's liver medicines are *Quassia, Chelidonium, Liquor calc. mur., Nux vom., Crocus,* and *Carduus,* though he does not reckon the last-named as solely an hepatic. These remedies have been already sufficiently considered, excepting *Crocus* and *Quassia,* and of this latter I have myself no experience, and will therefore pass it by. Of the former I will presently speak.

RADEMACHER ON THE INFLUENCE OF *Saffron* ON THE LIVER.

Crollius. in his treatise, *De signaturis internis rerum,* cites *Saffron* as a remedy for jaundice. Rade-

macher had been treating liver diseases with *Carduus*, and finding
the prevailing genius of disease
alter (which he recognized from
the fact that *Carduus* had ceased
to cure the then prevailing liver
affections), he began to test afresh
for the remedy, and believed he had
found in it *Quassia*.

A man of sixty years of age
came under his observation for a
painful chest affection, with fever,
cough, and bloody expectoration—
(we should now call such a case
pneumonia, broncho-pneumonia, or
pleuro-pneumonia, probably.)

The action of *Quassia* was fair,
but not so pronounced and rapid
as Rademacher was accustomed to,

and hence he concluded that he was not dealing with a real *Quassia* liver disease.

Patient took the *Aqua quassiæ* for a week with some obvious bene-fit, when, tiring of its taste, *Saffron* was added to colour and mask it. Result: rapid and complete cure.

Subsequent observations shewed that the curative virtue lay in the *Saffron*, and not in the *Quassia*.

DYSENTERIA HEPATIC CURED BY
Crocus.

Fever, colic, vomiting, rectal tenesmus, slimy, sanguineous, non-fœcal motions, easily and promptly cured with small doses of the tincture of *Saffron*, because dependent upon a primary affection of the liver curable by *Saffron*.

"In former years I should," says Rademacher, "have rushed into print in the medical journals and proclaimed *Saffron* as the greatest liver medicine extant, but since Paracelsus has broken my spectacles I see nature with my eyes alone, and it is now manifest to me that we cannot ascribe to any organ-remedy whatsoever absolute and unconditional curative power, but that the really clear and obvious revelation of the same depends upon the kind of the epidemic genius of disease that happens for the time-being to be prevailing."

Those who know their *Synden-ham* will appreciate this.

RADEMACHER'S CURE OF GALL-STONES.

Rademacher's observations are in all cases so reliable that I deem it a useful undertaking to give, in short, the gist of his experience of the medicinal cure of Gallstones.

Carduus, he maintains, is *facile princeps* in the attack; nothing equals it, he says. He was once enabled to recognise the presence of biliary calculi in the following extraordinary manner:—

An elderly man, who had formerly complained of heartburn, fulness, and regurgitation after food, was seized with violent colic, and, as all the abdominal remedies were without effect, he concluded that the abdominal affection was symptomatic of some other primarily diseased organ. He was sent for at an unusual hour to hear from the good man's wife that a bandage with a knot in it at once stopped the pain. From this he concluded that only a mechanical affection could be thus mechanically helped.

A slight and very peculiar feeling alone remained in the region of the gall bladder. Patient was treated during six months with Durand's remedy, and was thereby completely cured of his supposed stomachic affection and of his colic. He remained quite well for twelve years. Then, after this long interval, the stony guest again put an appearance, though under another guise. He again administered Durand's remedy whereupon the troubler ceased and came no more, the patient dying long after at a great age of senile marasm.

Rademacher relates how the symptoms of pleurisy and even of pneumonia may be really those of biliary calculi, and he instances the case of the wife, or rather widow of an admiral who was cured of an attack of gallstone colic with Durand's remedy by him, and, being seemingly well, travelled to Berlin, but fell ill of the same offection which was mistaken for pleurisy, and treated as such in the old antiphlogistic fashion with venesection and plasters, and under these the seventy-year old lady died.

Rademacher cites the case as a warning to the careless or inexperienced. He then remarks that *Sulphuric acid* has the power of stirring up biliary calculi to activity.

Of the tincture of *Carduus* in the attacks of gallstone colic he reccommends from 15 to 30 drops in a teacupful of water or milk five times a day.

Mixture of Oil of Terpentine and Sulphuric Æther, or Durand's Remedy.

Paracelsus says that the oil of turpentine was first discovered by the jatro-chemists, and he strongly recommends physicians to try the curative effects of the oil in diseased human organisms.

Rademacher remarks, however, that as a rule physicians are more concerned to gain over the patient-world by saying smooth thing to them than with the advancement of the healing art, and hence the recommendation was not followed and fell into oblivion.

Paracelsus affirms that turpentine with the right appropriate or organ remedies is helpful in all indurations.

Those who know of turpentine only that it is good for tapeworm, and that it, combined with æther, will dissolve gallstones, know but very little of its virtues.

He thus summarises: "All we can with certainty maintain is, that the symptoms which we ascribe to the presence of biliary calculi are not merely silenced by

12 -

turpentine in æther, but by its long continued use are got rid of so completely that patients remain thereafter free of their troubles forever, or, at any rate, for many years."

He finally remained true, after many trials, to a mixture of sixteen parts of *Spirit sulph. æth.*, and one of *Ol. tereb.*

And as to dose: one must begin gently and cautiously with ten, and, in the very sensitive, with five drops of the mixture in half a cupful of water three times a day, and the dose must be slowly or rapidly increased occording to the tolerance of each individual case.

At first there is often a little pain in the liver soon after the dose, lasting a few minutes. This he declares is desirable, but the dose must not be increased till this pain has not been felt for a few days. Then the urine must be watched, and as soon as the urine begins to get darker in colour (in which case the patient at the same time is apt to complain of an uncomfortable sensation in the epigastrium), the said mixture must be temporarily stopped and *Carduus* administered till the discomfort in the epigastrium has gone, and until the urine has again become clear and of the colour of light straw. And then the mixture is to be resumed, but in a small dose—smaller than it was when left off, and the dose is not to be too hastily again augmented.

CHRONIC ENLARGEMENT OF THE LIVER CURED BY *Podophyllum peltatum* 6[×].

In the month of June of the year 1883, a widow lady came under my observation for diarrhœa. It was clearly of hepatic nature, and patient felt as if she were sinking into the earth; icy cold feet; pains in the abdomen; has piles; last year nearly had jaundice. A physical examination revealed chronic enlargement of the liver; the pa-

tient looked ill, and in very ill-
health.

With an enlargement of the
liver, tenderness of the hepatic region, pains in the abdomen, piles,
diarrhœa, and evident *Angegriffen-
sein* of the organism, I think the
ordination of *Podophyllum pelt.* 6×
may be fairly called scientific; in
fact, I maintain that the prescription was demonstrably and strictly
scientific.

It cured the patient slowly—
seven weeks—surely, and permanently, and not only subjectively
but objectively, for her improved
appearance was very pronounced.

I often wonder in this age of science that its scientific spirit so much neglects the scientific therapeutics of Samuel Hahnemann, particularly as Hahneman has been so long dead. It cannot now make any difference to him! And faith! it makes no difference to me either

Then why do I stand up for homœopathy so persistently if it makes no difference to me?

Why, indeed?

Only one reason.

And what might that one reason be? Shall I confess, or let the black secret die with me?

Just this: *Homœopathy is true,
that's all.*

And if true, why do people sneer
at it?

Fools always do sneer at what
they do not understand.

PRACTICE OF MODERN FRENCH PHYSICIANS IN THE TREATMENT OF HEPATIC COLIC.

M. Germain Sée in "*La Médecine Moderne,*" *Nr.* 6, 1890, treats of this subject, and shows a distinct advance on the common treatment of hepatic colic.

He notes, that the *Salicylate of Sodium* is an excellent cholagogue; in watery solution the *Salicylate of Sodium* augments the biliary secretion, and particularly the *watery part of the bile.* And further, by a singular coincidence, this remedy, besides its action as

a cholagogue, has a powerful anal-
gesic action which is of prime
importance in the attack.

He insists that in prescribing
cholagogues great care should be
taken in dissolving them in an
ample quantity of fluid.

Rademacher was clearly of the
same view, for he gave each dose
of *Carduus* in a teacupful of fluid.

M. Sée speaks also with much
satisfaction of the free use of *Olive
Oil* in biliary attacks.

He considers purgatives contra-
indicated. He also condemns all
substances that lessen the biliary
secretion, such as the salts of

potassium, calomel, iron, copper, morphia, atropine, and strychnine,

But as M. Sée ignores the double and opposite actions of large and small doses, we can only regard him, in practical pharmacodynamics, as a half-educated man; and this, notwithstanding his pre-eminently leading position in the practice of modern medicine in France. But it is something to find anyone's practice addressed to the causes of the colic, rather than to silencing the pains, which are but effects, and which, being silenced, leave the morbid state of the sufferer as bad or even worse than it was before.

REMARKABLE CASE OF JAUNDICE
OF NINE YEARS' DURATION,
GALLSTONES OF LARGE SIZE.

I really finished writing this
small treatise on Liver Diseases
last autumn, and sent the MS. to
the printers, on the day the date of
which will be found at the foot of
my preface. In this same preface
mention is made of a case of
chronic jaundice of long duration,
which I then feared was hopelessly
incurable. This work has been
delayed at the printers until now,
owing to want of time on my part,
and moreover, I have latterly delayed it somewhat on purpose, and
in order that I may narrate the

before-mentioned case referred to in the preface, in which I reflect upon the treatment of the case followed by a distinguished representative of old-chool medicine.

I always hold that adverse criticism of co-practitioner's work should be in the abstract, because it is not in any sense a question of persons. I also hold that whosoever criticises the work of another adversely, the same is morally bound to point out a better, a more excellent way, if he knows one.

The plan followed by my predecessor in the treatment of this case was *to lull the pain* with morphia. Now, quite apart from the deteriorating influence of the drug (a question I do not propose here to discuss), it must be manifest that the pain arose from the gallstones: and the lulling influence of the morphia not only did not cure, or even tend to cure, but actually tended to prevent nature from helping herself.

The physician knew perfectly well that he only relieved the pain; he was quite conscious that it was in no sense a cure. "The thing," said he, "is incurable; the pain is therefore, the legitimate object of palliative treatment." And I quite agree that a physician may not stand by and see pain without taking effective measures for its relief.

But the patient's *life* comes *first*, not the pain; and therefore, here everything hinges upon the question of curability or non-curability. Assuming that the case was really and truly incurable by medical art, then, of course, the lulling of the pain by morphia was right and proper, and moreover imperatively demanded on the ground of humanity alone; and where physician cannot cure he is at least bound to relieve pain. I therefore attach no blame to this physician personally, his error lies in his scholastic conceptions of what are the actual possibilities of drugs in the direct art-cure of disease; and in the unquestioning belief that what he and his fellow-believers in school-physic know, covers the *entire* field of the known and of the knowable, in curative medicine.

Paracelsus is ridiculed and contemned; Rademacher is almost unknown in the wider sphere of medicine. Homœopathy is not within earshot at all, *i. e.*, in the spheres that are deemed orthodox. It seems very odd, but all that is best in medicine, in so far as it relates to the art of healing is . . . *out*side!

Paracelsus is *out*side; Rademacher is *out*side; Hahnemann is

*out*side; the physician who gave
morphia for the case under study
is . . . *in*side.

I will now go on to the case in
question by narrating that patient,
a married lady, mother of a family,
was brought to me by her husband
with some difficulty, owing to her
great weakness and loss of flesh.

I noted as follows:—Mrs X., 38
years of age, eleven years married,
mother of seven children, came
under my observation on Septem-
ber 29, 1890. During the past
three months intensely jaundiced,
and is given up as past all hope of
recovery.

During the past nine years her doctor has been giving her morphia to ease the pain in the right side, left side, and in the stomach, abdomen, and hypogastrium respectively. At the present time she takes about a dozen quarter-grain pills of morphia a day; she is emaciated to a painful degree. The spleen is very much hypertrophied, and extends across to the mesial line and inferiorly down to the crest of the ilium; in fact, it practically fill the left half of the abdomen. It is very tender, and the contours of the big spleen can not only be felt but readily seen, as it rises above the surface. The liver is only very moderately enlarged, about an inch and a half

beyond the ribs, towards the epi-
kastrium.

While I am examining her,
patient appears very weak and
faint, and hardly able to bear the
undressing. Her eyes are lustrous,
her tongue raw red. Urine is
scanty; loaded with bile; bowels
costive. The region of the gall-
bladder and ducts very tender, but
the greatest pain is in the pit of
the stomach. Catamenia always
scanty, and at present stopped.
The motions are without bile, and
moved with the very greatest difficulty. No appetite. In almost
constant distress from the agoni-
sing pains at the pit of the
stomach.

Patient had been twice vaccinated, and years ago had severe
ulceration of the womb, for which
she lay in bed for three months,
and during that period was six
times cauterised. The cauteriza-
tions, aided by many introvaginal
injections and much lying-up,
were followed by the disappearance
of said ulcerations.

I did not really know where to
begin at in this formidable case,
but in view of the severity of the
epigastric pain, jaundice, constipation, &c., I ordered *Hydrastis
Can.* φ, four drops in a tablespoonful of tepid water every four hours.
This was the last day of Septem-
ber, 1890.

October 6th.—The urine has begun to improve; it is more watery, and not quite so full of bile; the motions more natural, but the liver is very distinctly bigger than it was six days ago. I therefore feel justified in going on with the *Hydrastis*.

13th.—Patient's jaundiced skin is not quite so intensely black-yellow; the pain has *altered*. There is very distinct, though not great, improvement; for the first time for very very long her period is full and free, which has much relieved her. The spleen is a trifle smaller; the tongue dry and glazed.

I find on reference that a few doses of *Thuja* 30 were given intercurrently on the 6th instant. Continue with both *Hydrastis* φ and the *Thuja* 30.

20th.—There is no longer any pain in the region of the gall-bladder; patient complains of cold shivers; liver has gone down in size while the spleen is more swelled and very painful, and patient complains very much of chilliness.

℞. *Tc. Urticæ urentis* φ, seven drops in water three times a day.

27th.—No "spasms"; pains in the spleen worse; the spleen is, however, softer to the feel; liver larger. To alternate *Carduus mar.* φ with the *Urtica*, every three hours.

Nov. 3rd.—Spleen and liver both bigger, which I take to mean that they are being acted upon by the remedies, particularly as patient is not so chilly and is in less pain. Patient has never ceased to take about a dozen morphia pills every day; some days many more.

To continue with the *Carduus* and *Urtica*.

12th.—The jaundice is much worse; the pains in the region of the gall-bladder are atrocious. I try to persuade the patient to leave off the morphia, so as to give the remedies a chance, but she appeals to me not leave her unhelped in her agony; I could not resist, and so consented to the morphia pills being continued.

We had made a little progress in the case, but not much, and I therefore made a further and very careful survey of the ætiological history of the case, and came to the conclusion that the whole thing was of *uterine* ORIGIN.

As I have had a good deal of clinical experience of *Bursa pastoris*, tending to shew that it is a remedy specifically affecting the womb in like manner as *Chelidonium* does the liver, I at once determined to test for the right *appropriatum uteri*, as I conceive Paracelsus or Rademacher might have done.

I reasoned from the clinical data taken in historic sequence that the primary affection years ago was uterine, and the hepatic affection consecutive thereto, and starting therefrom. I saw clearly that the old ulcerated condition was at the bottom of it, or rather that was as far back as I could get for the present. For although the *cause* of the ulcers was presumably the *fons et origo mali*, yet the real disease *at present* to be grappled with was the jaundice, the gallstones, and the colic.

In this case getting rid of the primary constitutional cause would not necessarily have mended matters, therefore I started with *Bursa pastoris* Φ, five drops in warm water every five hours.

That was on the 12th, and by the 17th there was a very extra-ordinary change come over the face of the case; indeed it was at first blush almost incredible. There was much less jaundice, the liver had gone down in size almost to normality, and the spleen was fully an inch smaller. Moreover, there was no pain in the liver at all.

My inkling that the start of the disease of the biliary apparatus was in the womb being thus confirmed, indeed, rendered certain, I continued with the *Bursa* as before.

Nov. 24th.—Although there has

been no further spasms, there has not been any further progress; patient does not sleep so well; the liver has again begun to enlarge, and there is no further diminution in the size of the spleen. Still, I did not feel justified in leaving off with *Bursa*, and hence I alternated it with *Chelidonium* Φ.

December.—Patient was very ill, and everybody gave her up, excepting myself. I did not see my way out of the wood, but still I hold that the physician who gives up a case before the patient dies is on a par with the soldier who runs away from the enemy. So here, though I was absolutely alone in my view, I refused to surrender.

The bowels had ceased to act; there was more jaundice again, and patient could no longer rise from her bed.

I then gave *Euonymin* $3^{\times}$, six grains every two hours, just as a liver remedy. Under very great agony patient in the course of a week or two passed a handful of gallstones by the bowels, and her jaundice was gone!

A number of the largest were obtained from the stools, and on account of the great interest of the case I now present my readers with a photogravure of them, taken by Sprague, of London, and which gives them in their natural size.

I have shewn these biliary calculi to certain medical friends, and amongst them to Dr. Robert T. Cooper, of London, as a curiosity.

I should explain that these biliary calculi were very much larger than here represented when they were first passed, but their outer layers were friable, and were washed, picked, and rubbed off before the calculi were brought to me; it is really only the hard kernels of the calculi which are given in this photogravure.

Notwithstanding the disappearance of the jaundice, and the passage of the gallstones as just described, patient had got very low, and the spleen did not seem to be any better subjectively, and not much smaller, and there was no period.

Here I gave *Ceonothus Am.* 1, five drops in water four times a day.

15th.—Patient has had severe rigors, seemingly caused by the *Ceanothus*, which is therefore discontinued. She has no appetite, and the menstruation has not appeared.

To have *Pulsatilla* 1, three drops in water every three hours.

20th.—Liver nearly normal; has just menstruated; the spleen has

gone down a little; the entire abdomen very tender all over; has
again had an awful attack of gallstone colic, and passed a number
of stones, one very large. There
is still bile in the urine.

To have *Bursa pastoris* φ, and
Nux vom. 1.

29th.—Another attack of colic;
a further passage of biliary calculi
—three large ones; patient is low
and weak, and prefers death to so
much pain. It is to be remembered
that large numbers of morphia pills
are being taken all this time. To
relieve the effects of the passage of
the calculi, and the almost general
feeling of bruisedness and tender-

ness, I ordered *Bellis perennis* φ,
eight drops in water every four
hours.

1891, Jan. 12th.—Great general
improvement from the use of the
Bellis perennis, but her liver and
spleen are more swelled and greatly
distress her.

℞ *Trit* $3^\times$ *Cholesterin.* Six
grains dry on the tongue every
four hours.

19th.—Spleen and liver seem
larger than ever. No **jaund**ice,
however. No menses.

Five drops of *Pulsatilla* φ three
times a day.

14

26th.—Has normally menstruated; liver smaller; spleen very tender.

℞ *Bursa pastoris* Φ. Five drops in a tablespoonful of water three times a day.

Feb. 3rd.—Has passed some more calculi; region of gall duct very tender; no jaundice; urine normal; is gaining flesh; the spleen is very large.

℞ *Tr. Ceanothus Americanus* 1. Five drops in water every four hours.

13th.—There is further improvement; she feels better; is beginning to go about like other people, has passed one gallstone of small size, and a number of lumps of "sooty stuff." Feels that this medicine has done her much good.

Rep.

23rd—The spleen has gone down about one inch and three quarters; has menstruated again normally; is increasing in weight.

Rep.

March 16th.—By letter I am informed that the spleen is not so well; and that there is a good deal of pain in the right side again.

℞ *Trit.* 3× *Leptandrin.* Six grains dry on the tongue, three times a day.

14

31st.—No improvement from the *Leptandrin*, and generally not so well, though the jaundice is entirely a thing of the past, and she is now of a very clear white complexion, and getting no longer to appear to be particularly thin.

℞ *Bellis perennis* and *Bursa pastoris* in alternation.

April 15th—Liver, spleen, and womb are described as "all blown out;" much pain in the region of the gall bladder.

℞ *Puls.* and *Byronia.*

May 4th.—Patient is doing well; liver normal, or nearly so; spleen now only reaches half way down to the crest of the ilium, and is well defined. *Patient has now the old symptoms of ulceration of the* OS UTERI—*the forcible healing up of which started the whole thing years ago!*

And here I think I may resume, and conclude this already too long narration.

We see in this case the importance of Paracelsic organ-testing to find out the *point de départ* of the series of morbid phenomena; hepatics and splenics had no adequately curative action till the uterine medicine (*Bursa pastoris*) had touched the place of origin of the liver affection, and as soon as

this was done (see Notes under
date November 17th, 1890) immediate improvement began!

We have now cured the jaundice; the gallstones have been got
rid of through the natural ways;
the liver is well, and patient is
going about her business; and our
interest in the case IN THIS TREA-
TISE on "The Diseases of the
Liver" is at an end.

THREE MONTHS LATER.

August 10th, 1891.—Having this
day seen and carefully examined
this patient I am enabled to say
that she is in excellent health,
plump and pleasing, and equal to

and performing the usual duties of an English housewife with a large family.

PART III.

PART III.

The Diseases of the Liver

THE issue of a second edition of this treatise on Diseases of the Liver affords me an opportunity of adding somewhat to the clinical demonstrations already contained in Part II.

Particularly would I call attention to what is here related of the sphere of action of *Chelone glabra* of which no mention is made in the first edition, because I was, at the time of its issue, not clear on the subject. At this place I would also take the opportunity of pointing out the omission by Dr. Dudgeon of a very important point in regard to the clinical use of *Carduus mariæ*. Some time since Dr. Dudgeon translated and published in one of our journals some very important cases of pulmonary disease and coughs as cured by *Carduus*. The impression conveyed by this eminent writer's translation is that *Carduus* in these cases acted as a pulmonary remedy whereas the cases were really considered by their author as of *hepatic* origin: the pulmonary manifestations being consentaneous, or secondary to primary liver affections in all the cases narrated. This point is of the highest importance as Dr. Dudgeon's translations give one the impression that *Carduus* is a lung medicine which I think is entirely erroneous: the lung affections that are curable by *Carduus* have their starting point in a primary affection of the liver. All the clinical writers on *Carduus* with whose works I am acquainted are of this opinion, and Rademacher, the greatest of them all, is very clear and positive on the subject.* I will now relate a case of hepatic disease of great interest which had baffled some of the best physicians in London and which very clearly exemplifies the thera-

---

*I am very well aware that Dr. Dudgeon does not share in my organopathic views, but as translator he is bound to faithfully render the riginal.

peutic range of *Bellis perennis* and again of *Carduus mariæ*. It is one of:

ENLARGEMENT OF LIVER REMAIN-
ING FROM HEPATITIS AND
PERITONITIS.

The wife of the Vicar of St. B. brought a young lady, about 24 years of age, to me on February 20th, 1893, for considerable swelling of the abdomen and such severe varicosis of lower extremities that the patient had been confined to her couch for nearly a year. Patient had had thrombosis of the veins of her lower extremities repeatedly and the swelling in the right side of the abdomen dates

from a severe attack of peritonitis
and hepatitis. All idea of a cure
had been abandoned. Percussion
and palpitation revealed an enlargement of the left lobe of the
liver and a painful lump lying between the liver and the navel about
the size of a small fist. Glands in
the groins feel like marbles, lower
extremities large and unshapely,
clearly the remains of the original thrombosis. Inasmuch as the
whole series of phenomena—thrombosis, peritonitis, hepatitis—began
with getting a chill (cold, wet) six
years ago, I ordered my old friend
Bellis perennis ten drops in a tablespoonful of water night and morning.

March 20th.—Very greatly improved, indeed, lump nearly gone *and the lower extremities are now shapely ! !*

The left lobe of the liver however remaining enlarged, I ordered *Carduus mariæ* seven drops in water night and morning.

April 28th.—Patient at this date was walking about like other people, and the only thing that remained was a little transverse swelling of the liver and this was removed by a short course of *Chelone glabra.*

In the fall of the year 1893, a slight relapse occurred which was quickly righted by *Bellis perennis.*

The Vicar's wife was with me on October 15th, 1894, on another matter and mentioned incidentally that Jessie's cure had proved complete and lasting.

The common sunflower is an old horticultural as well as clinical friend of mine that has here and there helped me in splenic affections. Here I use it more as a liver remedy:—

Helianthus Annus AS A LIVER MEDICINE.

Altho' I regard the sunflower as specially a spleen medicine still it has a distinct action across from the spleen toward the liver and possibly it influences the liver also.

I have lately cured a stubborn case of a throbbing swelling in the pit of the stomach involving the left side of the liver and the spleen and the tissues lying between the two organs.

No defined epigastric tumours could be satisfactorily distinguished but the whole epigastric region was very tender on pressure and patient could not bend down without getting giddy and feeling much distress at the epigastrium. The particular interest in the case lay in the long duration of the ailment and the *pulsating epigastric mass.*

Patient took five drops of the matrix tincture of *Helianthus,* night and morning for some weeks when the only abnormal thing remaining was the very slight enlargement of the left lobe of the liver and for which he was put on *Chelone glabra.* The spleen was put right and also the epigastrium of which the pulsation ceased, together with the tenderness and distension and in view of the difficulties one encounters in dealing curatively with pulsating epigastric swellings I think this short narration worth penning and preserving.

I know of nothing in the way of diagnosis offering more difficulties and pit-falls than "pulsating tumours" in the abdomen, and indeed all abdominal tumours take a deal of diagnosing.

15

I will now invite my reader to a short yet closer consideration of an hepatic that is a comparatively new friend, viz·

Chelone Glabra—AN IMPORTANT HEPATIC.

I think I have discovered an important differential point for the scientific use of *Chelone glabra*.

A Commander in the Royal Navy, about two years ago, came under my observation for an enormous varix in the right groin, just on Poupart's ligament. The varix was about the size of a very small orange and the thing was certainly becoming alarming on account of the thinning of the wall of the dilated vein. And being in the bend of the groin it was almost impossible to apply mechanical support. The patient was a thoroughly healthy fellow and though I diagnosed him up and down and questioned him unto very weariness, still there was absolutely nothing findable beyond a slight enlargement of the left lobe of the liver. I first used *Chelidonium majus*. with some advantage, and under *Carduus mariæ* the varix certainly diminished somewhat, but under the remedy in question the varix disappeared and patient hastened off on active service. From this (and similar observations I have laid it down for my own future guidance that the *seat of action* of *Chelone glabra* is the left lobe of the liver and its *line of action* is in the direction of the navel, bladder and uterus. That this is really so the competent will have no difficulty in verifying whether *Chelone* acts upon the liver itself as a true hepatic I would not venture to affirm; perhaps it reduces the swellings of the left lobe of the liver by its action on the veins running up to the liver.

Many of the "New Remedies" have come and gone; *Chelone* has come to stay: its sphere of action is small, its action sharp and withal well defined

CASE OF RIGHT-SIDED VARICOCELE FROM ENLARGED LIVER, MUCH AMELIORATED BY *Chelone Glabra.*

A gentleman, who had long been under me, consulted me again in the spring of 1894 for varicocele of the right side. Casting about to find the primary dam I found the left lobe of the liver notably swelled, patient himself being however in capital health. There was besides the varicocele a moderate degree of varicosis of the large veins of the whole of the right leg. I prescribed *Chelone glabra,* five drops in a tablespoonful of water night and morning.

I did not hear from him for eleven months when he called to see me telling me he had gone on with the remedy steadily all the time as it seemed to be doing him good.

On examining him I found the varicocele had gone down about one-half and the varicosis of the leg had also notably diminished, so that he can now safely dispense with the elastic support. J was here led to prescribe *Chelone* because of its *line of action* from right to left and from above downwards.

The testimony afforded by this

case is very high indeed because
patient has been under me for
years for his varicosis with but
small benefit, and his being an
officer in the Royal Navy rendered
it very important that he should
have his varicosis mended. He is
not entirely cured now but the
amelioration is such that in his
own words "they (the authorities)
will let me go now on any expedi-
tion." I had before made use of a
number of vein medicines and constitutional remedies, but *Chelone*
alone did ten times more than they
all.

Carduus Mariæ AND *Chelone Glabra.*

There are cases of enlargement of the left lobe of the liver that are ameliorated by *Carduus mariæ*, and by *Chelone glabra* also, though not radically cured by either and these cases beautifully exemplify the limitations of the curative spheres of organ-remedies as I have more particularly dwelt upon in my work on "Diseases of the Spleen." The subject is so important that I will go into the matter at this place somewhat more in detail. It is a great help in the drug treatment of disease to be able to get clean-out constant indications for our remedies; and so it is very helpful to see where the remedial action certainly *leaves off* Now the curative sphere of organ-remedies stops *short of blood* diseases; they do *not reach* the diathesis, and they therefore do not cure, *e. g.*, Chronic Skin Diseases; skin diseases are commonly diathesic.

A gentleman of thirty years of age came under my observation for liver disease, skin disease, insomnia, depression of spirits and chronic diarrhœa tho', only thirty years of age, he has lost all his teeth from shrinking of the gums; they just fell out. His skin dis-

ease consisted in what I have else-
where called the *Sternal Patch*, the
liver affection in an enlargement
of the left lobe and for this I
ordered *Carduus mariæ*, six drops
in water, three times a day.   In a
short time he reported himself as
sleeping well and his spirits notably improved.   *Arsenicum* and
Thuja followed but no further improvement worth while mention-
ing, when, on June 13th, I prescribed *Chelone glabra* in the same
manner in which I had formerly
ordered *Carduus.*

July   13th.—" That   medicine
(*Chelone*) acted like a charm.

Patient remained well for a year
or so and then returned with the

old symptoms again—I have now come to the point of my case. *Carduus* was ordered as before. *Chelone* followed, but neither acted as formerly, that which a year before acted like a charm now acted not at all. The fact is in this case there exists a constitutional crasis quite away from the hepatic state, it is an organismic ailing and not merely one of the organ, and here I found it necessary to go in quest of the homœopathic simillimum, the simple homœopathic part-elective drug-effinity not sufficing. Clearly organ-remedies restore only tone and equable circulation in most instances but do not alter the organismic quality of the organ, nor do they cure any diathesic quality of the stroma of the organ.

In fine : Where the organ-ill comes from the organism and keeps on coming, the organ remedy is capable only of clearing the organ of its organismic soot, so to speak, for the time being; it is only while where the organ ailment is in and of the organ that the organ remedy is adequate. Also where the ailment is in and of the organ it is useless to attempt its cure with high dilutions affecting the whole organism: a localized organ disease calls for a localized organ remedy, just as a general diathesic organismic disease needs the homœopathic simillimum in some potency

sufficiently removed from its ma-
teriality. The degree of homœopathicity conditions the degree of
potency, the greater the degree of
of homœopathicity the greater
(higher) the potency and con-
versely. Hence it is that I use
mother tinctures in the organopathic states and ailments. Thus
even in the use of simple organ-
remedies of but small pathogenetic
powers, yet considerable local affinity, a few drops of the mother
tincture may act very perturbingly.
For instance the tincture of the
common marigold may be used in
5 or 10 drop doses with very slight
effect but let the homœopathicity
be a little greater than merely local

affinity and we get nausea, vomiting and abdominal distress.

Calendula AS A LIVER MEDICINE.

We find under *Calendula* "chilly hand." "He is easily frightened" —I have often used *Calendula* internally and gained the conviction that it has a certain beneficial influence upon scrofulous ulcers notably helping to make a nice scar. In liver affections I had not used it till Dr. Robert T. Cooper mentioned it to me in this regard, but he knew of no special indication for its use in preference to any other, and this is ever the great difficulty with organ-remedies, es-

pecially where the epidemic genius
of the disease is unknown, and, as
it so often is, unknowable; my
greatest help is to find out the
exact part of the organ or part, a
given remedy affects and this is
often quite sufficient.

The two symptoms, "chilly
hands" and "easily frightened,"
taken together and in conjunction
with liver troubles, would seem to
call for *Calendula*.

Case.—Mr. X., a singer of world-
wide fame, had been under me for
some months with much advan-
tages under hepatics and renal
remedies he greatly improved, but
did not get rid of his "cold hands"
and "I am so dreadfully nervous,

16

I am frightened at everything, sometimes I dare not enter a cab or carriage, and feel it to be absolutely impossible to face the audience and my indigestion is pretty bad and I have a great deal of heartburn."

At the left side of the liver, deep in, seemed the faulty part.

℞. *Calendula off. ϕ*, five drops in water, night and morning, was ordered and after a month of this I heard "Oh, I am getting on splendidly; the heartburn is gone, my digestion is better, my hands have quite lost that nasty cold feeling and my nerve is so much better, I am quite a different man."

I had formerly won this gentleman's confidence by materially improving his grand voice.

What with?

Thuja occidentalis 30.

Why given?

For Vaccinosis.

The number of people I have benefitted by *Thuja* 30 is really almost beyond belief; one dose of six globules every week is my rule.

Chelone Glabra in Hepatic Dropsy.

In a case of severe dyspnœa from hepatic dropsy *Chelone glabra* rendered me good service; the case was very complicated inasmuch as in addition to bradycardia, cirrhosis of the liver and Bright's disease of the kidneys there was seemingly a tumour lying between the liver and the navel: tense, tender and certainly of quite a different nature to the general ascitic swelling. By reason of its topographic position and in view of the line of action of *Chelone* as I have before pointed out, I gave five drops of

Chelone φ in a tablespoonful of water every four hours and in less than a fortnight the lump between liver and navel had quite disappeared, and simultaneously therewith also the cardiac dyspnœa. I say cardiac dyspnœa as it lay in its origin between the liver and the heart, I could not trace any direct influence of *Chelone* on either the heart or kidneys though both were much influenced by the removal of the obstructive mass between liver and navel.

Quassia AS A LIVER MEDICINE.

It is difficult to conceive of anything outside of one's own self and one's own experience and hence it comes to pass that I have never been quite able to realize that *Quassia* has any action on the liver worth while. *Und Doch.*

Very early in 1895 a gentlemen sent me a young man from Hampstead who had been in vain operated on in University College Hospital and thence discharged as incurable. Incurable at twenty years of age!

This young man informed me that he left University College

Hospital quite lately and showed me a long scar in the right axillary line where an incision would have enabled an exploration of the right kidney region, gall bladder and back of liver, which no doubt was the object of the operation. He himself stated that it was for stone in the right kidney but on reaching the kidney no stone could be found and so the wound was stitched up, and as soon as it had healed-up patient was discharged as incurable.

Patient complained of attacks of severe pain at the back of the liver —just where the fresh scar is seen —coming on with vomiting at any time, any day and in any weather;

these attacks average about one a
week and the pain once on will
last from one to three days. Has
been subject to these attacks for
five years and has had to give up
all work for long and is now much
reduced in health and strength.
The vomiting comes on whenever
he attempts to eat. As the attack
comes on he swells and seems very
tight in the girth. In the perpendicular the hepatic dulness goes
right up to the nipple. I put
patient at first on *Hydrastis Canadensis*, then on *Urtica urens*, then
on *Chelidonium majus* with the
sole difference that under the *Chelidonium* the dull percussion note
of the liver in the mammary line
was a trifle less.

On April 9th I ordered *Quassia tincture* Φ, five drops in water every four hours.

23d. There is very great improvement and the young man has quite a different look, his low whining complaining tone having given way to much greater mental and physical alertness, only one attack of pain. Rep.

May 7th. There have been two attacks of pain, but very much less severe and he feels much stronger.

To take the *Quassia* in five drop doses three times a day.

May 21st. Attacks are much less in severity and less frequent.

Patient has put on flesh, the previous dirty colour of the skin of his face has gone and given place to a clean, healthy looking face. Rep.

Remains under treatment so I am not able to say whether the *Quassia* is the real remedy in the case; but, assuming that it does no more than it has already accomplished, at any rate its record in the case is better than that of my allopathic friends at University College Hospital. So far as I see at present it is a case of neither liver nor kidney *merely*; but of the right supra-renal capsule, but into this dark continent we will now not penetrate.

INDEX.

PAGE.